STATISTICAL ASPECTS OF THE DESIGN AND ANALYSIS OF CLINICAL TRIALS

STATISTICAL ASPECTS
OF THE DESIGN
AND ANALYSIS OF
CLINICAL TRIALS

Brian S. Everitt
Institute of Psychiatry, London

Andrew Pickles
University of Manchester

Imperial College Press

ICP

Published by

Imperial College Press
57 Shelton Street
Covent Garden
London WC2H 9HE

Distributed by

World Scientific Publishing Co. Pte. Ltd.
P O Box 128, Farrer Road, Singapore 912805
USA office: Suite 1B, 1060 Main Street, River Edge, NJ 07661
UK office: 57 Shelton Street, Covent Garden, London WC2H 9HE

British Library Cataloguing-in-Publication Data
A catalogue record for this book is available from the British Library.

ISBN   1-86094-153-2

This book is printed on acid-free paper.

Printed in Singapore by Regal Press (S) Pte. Ltd.

PREFACE

According to Sir David Cox, the randomised controlled clinical trial is perhaps the outstanding contribution of statistics to 20th century medical research. Nowadays about 8000 such trials are undertaken annually in all areas of medicine from the treatment of acne to the prevention of cancer. Although the vast majority of these trials take place away from the glare of public interest, some deal with issues that are controversial enough to make even the popular press; an obvious example is the use of AZT for the treatment of AIDS.

There are many excellent books available which give comprehensive accounts of how clinical trials should be carried out and organised. Our aim is somewhat different; we attempt to give relatively concise descriptions of the more statistical aspects of the design and analysis of clinical trials, particularly those methods developed over the last decade or so. Topics discussed in this text include randomisation, interim analyses, sample size determination, the analysis of longitudinal data, Bayesian methods, survival analysis and meta-analysis. Many examples are included alongside some of the necessary technical material, the more difficult parts of which are confined to tables. An Appendix gives details of relevant software. We hope that our book will be useful to medical statisticians and others faced with the often difficult problems of designing and analysing clinical trials.

Our thanks are due to Dr Sophia Rabe-Hesketh and Dr Sabine Landau for reading the text and making many helpful suggestions, to Professor Elizabeth Kuipers for allowing us to use the economic data from her CBT trial in Chapter 4 and to Mrs Harriet Meteyard for help in compiling the references.

Brian S. Everitt and Andrew Pickles
London, 1999

Contents

CHAPTER 1

An Introduction to Clinical Trials

1.1. INTRODUCTION

Avicenna, an Arabian physician and philospher (980–1037), in his encyclopedic *Canon of Medicine*, set down seven rules to evaluate the effect of drugs on diseases. He suggested that a remedy should be used in its natural state, with uncomplicated disease, and should be observed in two 'contrary types of disease.' His *Canon* also suggested that the time of action and reproducibility of the treatment effect should be studied (Crombie, 1952; Meinert, 1986).

But for several centuries Avicenna's advice appears to have been largely ignored, with most ideas affecting choice of treatment depending largely on serendipity rather then planned experiments. Only in recent years (although see next section) has it become widely recognised that properly conducted *clinical trials*, which follow the principle of scientific experimentation provide the only reliable basis for evaluating the efficacy and safety of new treatments.

And just what constitutes a clinical trial? There are several possible definitions, but for our purposes the term will be used for any form of planned experiment designed to assess the most appropriate treatment of future patients with a particular medical condition, where the outcome in a group of patients treated with the test treatment are compared with those observed in a similar group of patients receiving a control treatment, and patients in both groups are enrolled, treated and followed over the same time period. The groups may be established through randomisation or some other method of assignment. The outcome measure may be the result of a laboratory test, a quality of life assessment, a rating of some characteristic or, in some cases, the death of a patient.

As a consequence of this somewhat restricted definition, comparative studies involving animals, or studies that are carried out *in vitro* using biological substances from man do not qualify as clinical trials. The definition also rules out detailed consideration of investigations involving *historical controls*.

1.2. A BRIEF HISTORY OF CLINICAL TRIALS

It is almost *de rigeur* in books on clinical trials to include a section tracing their history. Our book is no exception! Table 1.1 (taken from Meinert, 1986) lists some important dates in the development of such trials, the first of which relates to the often described experiment of James Lind carried out in 1747 while at sea on board the *Salisbury*. Bradford Hill (1962) gives the following quotation from Lind's account.

On the 20th May 1747, I took twelve patients in the scurvy, on board the Salisbury at sea. Their cases were as similar as I could have them. They all in general had putrid gums, the spots and lassitude, with weakness of their knees. They lay together in one place, being a proper apartment for the sick in the fore-hold; and had one diet in common to all, viz. water-gruel sweetened with sugar in the morning; fresh mutton broth often times for dinner; at other times puddings, boiled biscuit with sugar etc. And for supper, barley and raisins, rice and currants, sago and wine, or the like. Two of these were ordered each a quart of cider a day. Two others took twenty-five gutts of elixir vitriol three times a day, upon an empty stomach; using a gargle strongly acidulated with it for their mouths. Two others took two spoonfuls of vinegar three times a day, upon an empty stomach: having their gruels and their other food well acidulated with it, as also the gargle

Table 1.1. Historical Events in the Development of Clinical Trials.

Date	Author	Event
1747	Lind	Experiment with untreated control group (Lind, 1753)
1799	Haygarth	Use of sham procedure (Haygarth, 1800)
1800	Waterhouse	U.S.-based smallpox trial (Waterhouse, 1800, 1802)
1863	Gull	Use of placebo treatment (Sutton, 1865)
1923	Fisher	Application of randomisation to experimentation (Fisher and MacKenzie, 1923)
1931	—	Special committee on clinical trial created by the Medical Research Council of Great Britain (Medical Research Council, 1931)
1931	Amberson	Random allocation of treatment to groups of patients (Amberson *et al.*, 1931)
1937	—	Start of NIH grant support with creation of the National Cancer Institute (National Institutes of Health, 1981b)
1944	—	Publication of multicenter trial on treatment for common cold (Patulin Clinical Trials Committee, 1944)
1946	—	Promulgation of Nuremberg Code for Human Experimentation (Curran and Shapiro, 1970)
1962	Hill	Publication of book on clinical trials (Hill, 1962)
1962	Kefauver and Harris	Amendments to the Food, Drug and Cosmetic Act of 1938 (United States Congress, 1962)
1966	—	Publication of U.S. Public Health Service regulations leading to creation of Institutional Review Boards for research involving humans (Levine, 1981)
1967	Chalmers	Structure for separating the treatment monitoring and treatment administration process (Coronary Drug Project Research Group, 1973a)
1979	—	Establishment of Society for Clinical Trials (Society for Clinical Trials, Inc., 1980)
1980	—	First issue of *Controlled Clinical Trials*

(Taken with permission from Meinert, 1986.)

for their mouths. Two of the worst patients, with the tendons in the ham rigid (a symptom none of the rest had) were put under a course of sea-water. Of this they drank half a pint every day, and sometimes more or less as it operated, by way of a gentle physic. Two others had each two oranges and one lemon given them every day. These they eat with greediness, at different times, upon an empty stomach. They continued but six days under this course, having consumed the quantity that could be spared. The two remaining patients, took the bigness of a nutmeg three times a day of an electuary recommended by a hospital-surgeon, made of garlic, mustard-feed, rad. raphan, balsam of Peru, and gum myrr; using for common drink barley water well acidulated with tamarinds; by a decoction of which, with the addition of cremor tartar, they were greatly purged three or four times during the course. The consequence was, that the most sudden and visible good effects were perceived from the use of the oranges and lemons; one of those who had taken them, being at the end of six days fit for duty. The spots were not indeed at that time quite off his body, nor his gums sound; but without any other medicine, than a gargle of elixir vitriol, he became quite healthy before we came into Plymouth, which was on the 16th June. The other was the best recovered of any in his condition; and being now deemed pretty well, was appointed nurse to the rest of the sick.

In spite of the relative clear-cut nature of his findings, Lind still advised that the best treatment for scurvy involved placing stricken patients in 'pure dry air.' No doubt the reluctance to accept oranges and lemons as treatment for the disease had something to do with their expense compared to the 'dry air' treatment. In fact it was a further 40 years before the British Navy supported lemon juice for the crews of its ships at sea; once again the question of cost quickly became an issue with lemons being substituted by limes, condemming the British sailor to be referred to for the next two hundred years as 'limeys'.

Most of the early experiments involved arbitrary, nonsystematic schemes for assigning patients to treatments, such as that described by Lind. The concept of randomisation as a method for treatment assignment was first introduced by Fisher and the first trial with a properly randomised control group was for streptomycin in the treatment of pulmonary tuberculosis (see Medical Research Council, 1948, and Armitage, 1983). But not all clinicians were convinced of the need for such trials — the following is taken from a letter published in a medical journal of the day, attacking a proposed trial for the treatment of depression:

There is no psychiatric illness in which bedside knowledge and long clincal experience pays better dividends; and we are never going to learn about how to treat depressions properly from double blind sampling in an MRC statistician's office.

Since World War II, the clinical trial has evolved into a standard procedure in the evaluation of new drugs. Its features include the use of a control group of patients that do not receive the experimental treatment, the random allocation of patients to the experimental or control group, and the use of blind or masked assessment so that neither the researchers nor the patients know which patients are in either group at the time the study is conducted. The clinical trial nicely illustrates the desire of modern democratic society to justify its medical choices on the basis of the objectivity inherent in statistical and quantitative data.

1.3. TYPES OF CLINICAL TRIAL

Clinical trials can take a variety of different forms. All however are *prospective* with observations being made over a period of time after treatment allocation. Perhaps the most common design for a clinical trial is the fixed sample size *parallel groups* design with random allocation of patients to treatment, rather than some larger randomisation unit such as family, hospital, ward, community, etc. One problem with such a design occurs when patients vary so much in their initial disease state and in their response to therapy that large numbers of patients may be needed to estimate reliably the magnitude of any treatment difference. A more precise treatment comparison might be achieved by using a *cross-over* design in which each patient receives more than one treatment. A simple example is the 2×2 cross-over design in which one group of patients receive two treatments, A and B, in the order AB, another group in the order BA, with patients being randomly allocated to the two groups. Clearly such a design is only suitable for chronic conditions in which there is the limited objective of studying the patient's response to relatively short periods of therapy. The design and analysis of cross-over trials is more than adequately dealt with in Jones and Kenward (1989) and Senn (1993), and so will not be considered in any detail in this text.

The majority of randomised, placebo-controlled clinical trials have focussed on one drug at a time although this does not match up with clinical practice where it is rarely sufficient to consider only a single treatment for a condition. Questions about the effects of combinations of treatments can never be resolved by the simple parallel groups design in which an active treatment is compared with a placebo; consequently, some investigators have proposed *factorial designs* in which several treatments are considered simultaneously. Lubsen and Pocock (1994), for example, describe a trial in which patients were simultaneously randomised to each of three active treatments or their respective controls in a $2 \times 2 \times 2$ factorial arrangement. The claim made for the trial is that it provides three answers for the price of one (see Collins, 1993). As Lubsen and Pocock point out, this claim is only justified if it can safely be assumed that there is no evidence of any *interaction* between the three treatments. Lack of interaction implies that the effect of the treatments are additive on some particular scale expressing the effects of each treatment. Lubsen and Pocock are sceptical about whether interactions can often be dismissed *a priori*; if they cannot, then factorial designs will require larger sample sizes to achieve the same power as a parallel groups design. Their conclusion is that such designs are most appropriate for assessing therapeutic combinations when possible interactions are actually of primary interest. Some consideration of such studies is given in Holtzmann (1987) and Berry (1990).

The pharmaceutical industry uses a well-established taxonomy of clinical trials involving drug therapy, in which the categories can, according to Pocock (1983), be described as follows:

Phase I Trials: Clinical Pharmacoloy and Toxicity

These first experiments in man are primarily concerned with drug safety, not efficacy, and hence are usually performed on healthy, human volunteers, often pharmaceutical company employees. The first objective is to determine an acceptable single drug dosage (i.e. how much drug can be given without causing serious side-effects). Such information is often obtained from *dose-escalation* experiments, whereby a volunteer is subjected to increasing doses of the drug according to a predetermined schedule. Phase I will also include studies of drug metabolism and bioavailability and later, studies of multiple doses will be undertaken to determine appropriate dose schedules for use in phase II. After studies in normal volunteers, the initial trials in patients will also be of phase I type. Typically, phase I studies might require a total of around 20–80 subjects or patients. The general aim of such studies is to provide a relatively clear picture of a drug, but one that will require refinement during phases II and III.

Phase II Trials: Initial Clinical Investigation for Treatment Effect

These are fairly small-scale investigations into the effectiveness and safety of a drug, and require close monitoring of each patient. Phase II trials can sometimes be set up as a screening process to select out those relatively few drugs of genuine potential from the larger number of drugs which are inactive or over-toxic, so that the chosen drugs may proceed to phase III trials. Seldom will phase II go beyond 100–200 patients on a drug. The primary goals of phase II trials are:

- to identify accurately the patient population that can benefit from the drug,

- to verify and estimate the effectiveness of the dosing regimen
determined in phase I.

Phase III Trials: Full-scale Evaluation of Treatment

After a drug is shown to be reasonably effective, it is essential
to compare it with the current standard treatment(s) for the same
condition in a large trial involving a substantial number of patients.
To some people the term 'clinical trial' is synonymous with such a
full-scale phase III trial, which is the most rigorous and extensive
type of scientific clinical investigation of a new treatment.

Phase IV Trials: Postmarketing Surveillance

After the research programme leading to a drug being approved
for marketing, there remain substantial enquiries still to be undertaken as regards monitoring for adverse effects and additional large-
scale, long-term studies of morbidity and mortality.

This book will be largely concerned with phase III trials. In order to accumulate enough patients in a time short enough to make a
trial viable, many such trials will involve recruiting patients at more
than a single centre (for example, a clinic, a hospital, etc.); they
will be *multicentre trials*. The principal advantage of carrying out
a multicentre trial is that patient accrual is much quicker so that
the trial can be made larger and the planned number of patients can
be achieved more quickly. The end-result should be that a multicentre trial reaches more reliable conclusions at a faster rate, so that
overall progress in the treatment of a given disease is enhanced.

Recommendations over the appropriate number of centres varies;
on the one hand, rate of patient acquisition may be completely inadequate when dealing with a small number of centres, but with a large
number (20 or more) potential practical problems (see Table 1.2)
may quickly outweigh benefits. There also be other problems involving the *analysis* of multi-centre trials. It is likely, for example, that

Table 1.2. Potential Problems with Multicentre Trials.

- The planning and administration of any multicentre trial is considerably more complex than in a single centre,
- Multicentre trials are very expensive to run,
- Ensuring that all centres follow the study protocol may be difficult,
- Consistency of measurements across centres needs very careful attention,
- Motivating all participants in a large multicentre trial may be difficult,
- Lack of clear leadership may lead to a degeneration in the quality of a multicentre trial.

the true treatment effect will not be identical at each centre. Consequently there may be some degree of treatment-by-centre interaction and various methods have been suggested for dealing with this possibility. Details are available in Jones *et al.* (1998), Gould (1998) and Senn (1998).

1.4. ETHICS OF CLINICAL TRIALS

Since the time of Hippocrates, Western physicians have taken an oath in which they swear to protect their patients 'from whatever is deleterious and mischievous.' Unfortunately such an oath has not managed to stop many damaging therapies being given or to lessen the persistence of barbarous practices such as copious blood-letting. Even the most powerful members of society were vulnerable to the ill-informed, if well-intentioned physician, as the following account of the treatment of the dying Charles II demonstrates:

At eight o'clock on Monday morning of February 2, 1685, King Charles II of England was being shaved in his bedroom. With a sudden cry he fell backward and had a violent convulsion. He became unconscious, rallied once or twice, and after a few days, died. Doctor Scarburgh, one of the twelve or fourteen physicians called to treat the stricken king, recorded the efforts made to cure the patient. As the first step in treatment the king was bled to the extent of a pint from a vein in his right arm. Next his shoulder was cut into and the incised area was 'cupped' to suck out an additional eight ounces of blood. After this, the drugging began. An emetic and purgative were administered, and soon after a second purgative. This was followed by an enema containing antimony, sacred bitters, rock salt, mallow leaves, violets, beetroot, camomile flowers, fennel seed, linseed, cinnamon, cardamom seed, saphron, cochineal, and aloes. The enema was repeated in two hours and a purgative given. The king's head was shaved and a blister raised on his scalp. A sneezing powder of hellebore root was administered and also a powder of cowslip flowers 'to strengthen his brain.' The cathartics were repeated at frequent intervals and interspersed with a soothing drink composed of barley water, liquorice, and sweet almond. Likewise white wine, absinthe, and anise were given, as also were extracts of thistle leaves, mint, rue, and angelica. For external treatment a plaster of Burgundy pitch and pigeon dung was applied to the king's feet. The bleeding and purging continued, and to the medicaments were added melon seeds, manna, slippery elm, black cherry water, an extract of flowers of lime, lily of the valley, peony, lavender, and dissolved pearls. Later came gentian root, nutmeg, quinine and cloves. The king's condition did not improve, indeed it grew worse, and in the emergency forty drops of extract of human skull were administered to allay convulsions. A rallying dose of Raleigh's antidote was forced down the king's throat; this antidote contained an enormous number of herbs and animal extracts. Finally bezoar stone was given. "Then", said Scarburgh, "Alas! after an ill-fated night his serene majesty's strength seemed exhausted to such a degree that the whole assembly of physicians lost all hope and became despondent; still so as not to appear to fail in doing their duty in any detail, they brought into play the most active cordial." As a sort of grand summary to this pharmaceutical debauch, a mixture of Raleigh's antidote, pearl julep, and ammonia was forced down the throat of the dying king.

Ethical issues in medicine in general and clinical trials in particular are clearly of great importance and present a potential minefield especially for two statisticians more involved and perhaps more interested in the pragmatic problems of the analysis of the data generated in such trials. Nonetheless, along with all staff involved in trials, the statistician must share in the general responsibility for the ethical conduct of a trial. And there are in addition some areas of trial conduct where the statistician needs to take particular responsibility for ensuring that both the proposed and actual conduct of the trial are appropriate.

A central ethical issue often identified with clinical trials is that of randomisation. Randomised controlled trials are now widely used in medical research. Two recent examples from the many trials undertaken each year include:

- A multicentre study of a low-protein diet on the progression of chronic renal failure in children (Wingen *et al*; 1997),
- A study of immunotherapy for asthma in allergic children (Adkinson Jr. *et al.*, 1997).

Random allocation gives all subjects the same chance of receiving each possible treatment (although see Chapter 2). Randomisation serves several purposes; it provides an important method of allocating patients to treatments free from personal biases and it ensures a firm basis for the application of significance tests and most of the rest of the statistical methodology likely to be used in assessing the results of the trial. Most importantly, randomisation distributes the effects of concomitant variables, both measured and unobserved (and possibly unknown), in a chance, and therefore, impartial fashion amongst the groups to be compared. In this way, random allocation ensures a lack of bias, making the interpretation of an observed group difference largely unambiguous — its cause is very likely to be the different treatments received by the different groups.

Unfortunately, however, the idea that patients should be randomly assigned to treatments is often not appealing to many clinicians nor to many of the individuals who are prospective participants in a trial. The reasons for their concern are not difficult to identify. The clinician faced with the responsibility of restoring the patient to health and suspecting that any new treatment is likely to have advantages over the old, may be unhappy that many patients will be receiving, in her view, the less valuable treatment. The patient being recruited for a trial, having been made aware of the randomisation component, might be troubled by the possibility of receiving an 'inferior' treatment.

Few clinicians would argue against the need for the voluntary consent of subjects being asked to take part in a trial, but the amount of information given in obtaining such consent might be a matter for less agreement. Most clinicians would accept that the subject must be allowed to know about the randomisation aspect of the trial, but how many would want to go as far as Berry (1993) in advising the subject along the following lines?

I would like you to participate in a randomised trial. We will in effect flip a coin and give you therapy A if the coin comes up heads and therapy B if it comes up tails. Neither you or I will know what therapy you receive unless problems develop. [After presenting information about the therapies and their possible side-effects:] No one really knows what therapy is better and that is why we're conducting this trial. However, we have had some experience with both therapies, including experience in the current trial. The available data suggest that you will live an average of five months longer on A than on B. But there is substantial variability in the data, and many people who have received B have lived longer than some patients on A. If I were you I would prefer A. My probability that you live longer on A is 25 per cent.

Your participation in this trial will help us treat other patients with this disease, so I ask you in their name. But if you choose not to participate, you will receive whichever therapy you choose, including A or B.

Berry's suggestion as to how to inform subjects considering taking part in a clinical trial highlights the main ethical problem in such a study, namely the possible conflict between trying to ensure that each individual patient receives the treatment most beneficial for his/her condition, and evaluating competing therapies as efficiently as possible so that all future patients might benefit from the superior treatment. The great dilemma of clinical trials is that if each patient is treated as well as possible, patients as a whole are not. Lellouch and Schwartz (1971) refer to the problem as competition between *individual* and *collective* ethics. Pocock (1983) suggests that each clinical trial requires a balance between the two. The prime motivation for conducting a trial involves future patients, but individuals involved in the trial have to be given as much attention as possible without the trial's validity being destroyed. Naturally the clinician's responsibility to patients during the course of a trial are clear; if the patient's condition deteriorates, the ethical obligation must always and entirely outweigh any experimental requirements. This obligation means that whenever a physician thinks that the interest of a patient are at stake, she must be allowed to treat the patient as she sees fit. This is an absolutely essential requirement for an ethically conducted trial, no matter what complications it may introduce into the final analysis of the resulting data.

Clearly the ethical issues will be of greater concern in trials where the condition being treated is extremely serious, possibly even life threatening, than when it is more mild. The problems that can arise in the former situation are well illustrated by the history of the trials of AZT as a therapy for AIDS. When such trials were first announced there was a large, vocal lobby against testing the drug in a controlled clinical trial where necessarily some patients would receive an 'inferior treatment'. Later, however, when the severity of some side effects was identified and the long term effectiveness of the drug in doubt, an equally vocal lobby called for AZT treatment to be abandoned. Expanding networks of 'support groups' makes these problems increasingly likely.

If randomisation is the first priority in an acceptable clinical trial, *blinding* comes a close second. The fundamental idea of blinding is that the trial patients, the people involved with their management and those collecting clinical data from studies, should not be influenced by knowledge of the assigned treatment. Blinding is needed to prevent the possibility of bias arising from the patient, the physician and in evaluation. There are a number of levels of blinding of which the two most important are:

- *Single-blind*: Usually used for the situation in which the patient is unaware of which treatment he or she is receiving.
- *Double-blind*: Here both the patient and the investigator are kept blind to the patient's treatment. For many trials this is the arrangement of choice.

In drug trials blinding is usually relatively easy to arrange but the blinding of physical treatments, for example, surgical procedures, is often more difficult.

The randomised double-blind controlled trial is the 'gold-standard' against which to judge the quality of clinical trials in general. But such trials are still misunderstood by many clinicians and questions about whether or not they are ethical persist. One of the problems identified by Bracken (1987), is that doctors are frequently reluctant to accept their uncertainty about much of what they practice. Bracken concludes that when doctors *are* able to admit to themselves and their patients uncertainty about the best action, then no conflict exists between the roles of the doctor and the statistician. In such circumstances it cannot be less ethical to choose a treatment by random allocation within a controlled trial than to choose by what happens to be readily available, hunch, or what a drug company recommends. The most effective argument in favour of randomised clinical trials is that the alternative, practising in complacent uncertainty, is worse. All those points are nicely summarised in the following quotation from Sir George Pickering, made when President of the Royal Society of Medicine in 1949, in response to the charge that the clinical trial constituted experimentation on patients:

All therapy is experimentation. Because what in fact we are doing is to alter one of the conditions, or perhaps more than one, under which our patient lives. This is the very nature of an experiment, because an experiment is a controlled observation in which one alters one or more variables at a time to try to see what happens. The difference between haphazard therapy and a controlled clinical trial is that in haphazard therapy we carry out our experiments without design on our patients and therefore our experiments are bad experiments from which it is impossible to learn. The controlled clinical trial merely means introducing the ordinary accepted criteria of a good scientific experiment.

Further convincing *empirical* arguments in favour of the double-blind controlled clinical trial are provided by the work of Chalmers *et al.* (1977) and Sacks *et al.* (1983) who provide evidence that nonrandomised studies yield larger estimates of treatment effects than studies using random allocation (see Table 1.3), estimates that are very likely biased; and Schulz *et al.* (1995), who demonstrate that trials in which concealment of treatment allocation was either

Table 1.3. Results from Randomised and Historical Control Trials in Six Areas.

| | Randomised Trials | | Historical Control Trials | |
| | New treat. | New treat. | New treat. | New treat. |
Therapy	effective	ineffective	effective	ineffective
Coronary artery surgery.	1	7	16	5
Anticoagulants for acute myocardial infarction.	1	9	5	1
Surgery for oesophaeal varices.	0	8	4	1
Flurouracil (5-FU) for colon cancer.	0	5	2	0
BCG immunotherapy for melanoma.	2	2	4	0
Diethylstilbesterol for habitual abortion.	0	3	5	0

(Taken from Sacks *et al.*, 1983.)

inadequate or unclear (i.e., were not double-blind), also yielded larger (biased) estimates of treatment effects.

There are a number of other ethical issues in clinical trials which relate directly to one or the other of the statistical aspects of design and analysis; an example is determining the appropriate sample size by means of a power analysis — using too small or too large a sample would be unethical, a point that will be taken up in more detail in the next chapter.

1.5. CLINICAL TRIAL PROTOCOLS

All clinical trials begin with a protocol which serves as a guide for the conduct of the trial. The protocol must describe in a clear and unambiguous manner how the trial is to be performed so that all the investigators are familiar with the procedures to be used. The protocol must summarise published work on the study topic and use the results from such work to justify the need for the trial. If drugs are involved, then pertinent pharmacological and toxicity data should be included. The purpose of the trial and its current importance need to be described in clear and concise terms; hypotheses that the trial is designed to test need to be clearly specified and the population of patients to be entered into the trial fully described. The protocol must specify the treatments to be used; in particular, for drug studies, the dose to be administered, the dosing regimen, and the duration of dosing all need to be listed. Details of the randomisation scheme to be adopted must be made explicit in the protocol along with other aspects of design such as control groups, blinding, sample size determination and the number of interim analyses planned (if any). Although it is important that investigators adhere to the protocol, mechanisms need to be in place for making changes if the need arises. If changes are made, then they must be well documented.

1.6. SUMMARY

The controlled clinical trial has become one of the most important tools in medical research and investigators planning to undertake such a trial have no shortage of excellent books to which to turn for advice and information. But unlike the many other books dealing with clinical trials, this text is primarily concerned with the *statistical* issues of certain aspects of their design (Chapters 2 and 3) and, in particular, their analysis (Chapters 4 to 10), rather than their day-to-day organisation. This restriction will enable us to give fuller accounts of some recently developed methods that may be particularly useful for the type of data often generated from clinical trials. Some details of the software available that implements the methods described will be given in the Appendix.

Treatment Allocation, the Size of Trials and Reporting Results

2.1. INTRODUCTION

The design and organisation of a clinical trial generally involves a considerable number of issues. These range from whether it is appropriate to mount the trial at all, to selection of an appropriate outcome measure. Some of these issues will be of more concern to statisticians than others. Three of these: 1) allocating subjects to treatment groups; 2) deciding the size of the trial, i.e., how many subjects should be recruited; and 3) how results should be reported, will be discussed in this chapter.

2.2. TREATMENT ASSIGNMENT METHODS

One of the most important aspects of the design of a clinical trial is the question of how patients should be allocated to the various treatments under investigation. As Silverman (1985) put it:

How is the impossible decision made to choose between the accepted standard treatment and the proposed improved approach when a fellow human being must be assigned to one of the two (or more) treatments under test? Despite the most extensive pre-clinical studies, the first human allocation of a powerful treatment is largely a blind gamble and it is perhaps not surprising that so much has been written on the most appropriate fashion to allocate treatments in a trial.

Most of the early clinical experiments involved arbitary, nonsystematic schemes for assigning patients to treatments (see, for example, the description of Lind's experiment in Chapter 1). The concept of randomisation as a device for treatment assignment was introduced by Fisher in the 1920s (all-be-it in the context of agricultural experimentation). Randomised trials have been in existence since the 1940s but only in the last 10 or 20 years have they gained widespread acceptance. Possible ethical objections to randomisation were mentioned in Chapter 1, and many alternative methods of allocation have been suggested, the defficiencies of most of which are well documented in, for example, Pocock (1983). The main competitor to randomisation is the use of *historical controls*; all suitable patients receive the new treatment and their outcomes are compared with those from the records of patients previously given the standard treatment. Although there are considerable problems with the use of such controls (see Table 2.1), it has now become more widely recognised that they do have a role to play (see, for example, Simon, 1982),

Table 2.1. Problems with Historical Control Trials.

- Past observations are unlikely to relate to a precisely similar group of patients
- The quality of information extracted from the historical controls is likely to be different (probably inferior), since such patients were not intially intended to be part of the trial
- Patients given a new, and as yet, unproven treatment, are likely to be far more closely monitored and receive more intensive ancillary care than historical controls receiving the orthodox treatment in a routine manner
- For the reasons listed, studies with historical controls are likely to exaggerate the value of a new treatment (see Table 1.3).

particularly in providing the data on innovative treatments which might support further investigation in a randomised trial. Some advantages of historical control studies, particularly in cancer trials, listed by Gehan (1984) are:

- historical control studies can cost less than half as much as randomised studies with comparable sample sizes,
- there may be many more control patients available historically than concurrently,
- a clinician who believes (however weakly) that the experimental therapy is better than the control faces no ethical dilemma in admitting patients for treatment,
- patients are more apt to enlist for a study in which treatment assignment is not randomised.

But in this text our major concern is with *properly* randomised trials. The qualifier is needed here, since the acceptance of the principle of randomisation remains only a starting point in the execution of a trial. If the randomisation is not performed correctly in practice, then there is every danger that the trial could suffer from the same biases that are generally suspected in a trial not involving randomisation.

Randomisation in a two-group study might appear to be simply a matter of repeatedly tossing a coin in order to decide which of the two treatments each patient should receive, and indeed, in some circumstances this may be all that is needed. There are, however, other more complex randomisation schemes designed to achieve various objectives. We begin, though, with a few comments about the simple 'coin tossing' type of randomisation process. (Although we shall concentrate largely on trials in which the unit of randomisation is the individual patient, it is important to note that there are trials in which, for example, complete families are randomised to the various treatments to be compared. Such trials may need special methods of analysis as we shall mention later.)

2.2.1.   Simple Randomisation

For a randomised trial with two treatments, A and B, the basic concept of tossing a coin over and over again and allocating a patient to A if a head appears and B if the coin shows tails, is quite reasonable, but is rarely if ever used in practice. Instead, a randomisation list is constructed using a published table of random numbers or, more usually, a computer-based recognised pseudo-random number generator. The entries in this list can then be used one at a time as patients are recruited to the trial. (In a multicentre trial, each centre should have its own randomisation schedule so as to avoid treatment-centre confounding.)

The advantage of such a simple method is that each treatment assignment is completely unpredictable and in the long run the number of patients allocated to each treatment is unlikely to differ greatly. In the long run, however, implies a greater number of patients than are recruited to many clinical trials and it is of some interest to

Table 2.2. Possible Imbalance in Simple Randomisation with Two Treatments.

Shows the difference in treatment numbers (or more extreme) liable to occur with probability at least 0.05 or at least 0.01 for various trial size.

Total Number of Patients	Difference in Numbers	
	Probability ≥ 0.05	Probability ≥ 0.01
10	2:8	1:9
20	6:14	4:16
50	18:32	16:34
100	40:60	37:63
200	86:114	82:118
500	228:272	221:279
1000	469:531	459:541

(Taken with permission from Pocock, 1983.)

consider the chance of possible imbalance of patient numbers in the two groups. Table 2.2 (taken from Pocock, 1983), illustrates the differences in treatment numbers that may occur with probability greater than 0.05 and 0.01. For a trial with 20 patients, for example, the chance of four being allocated to one treatment and 16 to the other is greater than 0.01. Although this chance might be regarded as fairly small, the resulting imbalance would be of grave concern to most investigators, typically resulting in a study of much lower power than that expected from an even allocation of subjects (although see Section 2.2.5). Consequently, it is often desirable to restrict randomisation to ensure similar treatment numbers throughout the trial. (Although see later for situations when *unequal* group sizes may be a sensible feature of the design.) Several methods are available for achieving balanced group sizes of which the most commonly used is *blocked randomisation*.

2.2.2. Blocked Randomisation

This method introduced by Hill (1951), and also known as *permuted block randomisation*, guarantees that at no time during randomisation will the imbalance be large and that at certain points the number of subjects in each group will be equal. The essential feature of this approach is that *blocks* of a particular number of patients are considered and a different random ordering of treatments assigned in each block; the process is repeated for consecutive blocks of patients until all have been randomised. For example, with two treatments (A and B), the investigator may want to ensure that after every sixth randomised subject, the number of subjects in each treatment group is equal. Then a block of size 6 would be used and the process would randomise the order in which three As and three Bs are assigned for every consecutive group of six subjects entering the trial. There are 20 possible sequences of 3As and 3Bs, and one of these is chosen at random, and the six subjects are assigned accordingly. The process is repeated as many times as possible. When six patients are enrolled, the numerical balance between treatment A and treatment B is equal and the equality is maintained with the enrollment of the 12th, 18th, etc., patient.

Freidman, Furberg and DeMets (1985) suggest an alternative method of blocked randomisation in which random numbers between 0 and 1 are generated for each of the assignments within a block, and the assignment order then determined by the ranking of these numbers. For example, with a block of size six in the two treatment situation, we might have:

Assignment	Random Number
A	0.112
A	0.675
A	0.321
B	0.018
B	0.991
B	0.423

This leads to the assignment order BAABAB.

In trials that are not double-blind, one potential problem with blocked randomisation is that at the end of each block an investigator who keeps track of the previous assignments could predict what the next treatment would be. This could permit a bias to be introduced. The smaller the block size, the greater is the risk of the randomisation becoming predictable. For this reason, repeated blocks of size two should *not* be used. A required means of reducing the problem is by varying the size of consecutive sets. A random order of block size makes it very difficult to determine the next assignment in a series.

The great advantage of blocking is that balance between the number of subjects is guaranteed during the course of the randomisation. The number in each group will never differ by more than

$b/2$, where b is the size of the block. This can be important for two reasons. First if enrollment in a trial takes place slowly over a period of months or even years, the type of patient recruited for the study may change during the entry period (temporal changes in severity of illness, for example, are not uncommon), and blocking will produce more comparable groups. A second advantage of blocking is that if the trial should be terminated before enrollment is completed because of the results of some form of *interim analysis* (see Chapter 3), balance will exist in terms of the number of subjects randomised to each group.

2.2.3. Stratified Randomisation

One of the objectives in randomising patients to treament groups is to achieve between group comparability on certain relevant patient characteristics usually known as *prognostic factors*. Measured prior to randomisation, these are factors which it is thought likely will correlate with subsequent patient response or outcome. As mentioned in Chapter 1, randomisation tends to produce groups which are, on average, similar in their entry characteristics, both known and unknown. The larger a trial is, the less chance there will be of any serious non-comparability of treatments groups, but for a small study there is no guarantee that all baseline characteristics will be similar in the two groups. If prognostic factors are not evenly distributed between treatment groups, it may give the investigator cause for concern, although methods of statistical analysis such as *analysis of covariance* exist which allow for such lack of comparablity (see later chapters). *Stratified randomisation* is a procedure which helps to achieve comparability between the study groups for a chosen set of prognostic factors. According to Pocock (1983), the method is rather like an insurance policy in that its primary aim is to guard against the unlikely event of the treatment groups ending up with some major difference in patient characteristics.

The first issue to be considered when stratified randomisation is contemplated, is which prognostic factors should be considered. Experience of earlier trials may be useful here. For example, Stanley (1980) carried out an extensive study of prognostic factors for survival in patients with inoperable lung cancer based on 50 such factors recorded for over 5000 patients in seven trials. He showed that performance status, a simple assessment of the patient's ability to get around, was the best indicator of survival. Weight loss in the last six months and extent of disease also affected survival. These three factors would, consequently, be those to account for in any future trial.

When several prognostic factors are to be considered, a stratum for randomisation is formed by selecting one subgroup from each of them (continuous variables such as age are divided into groups of some convenient range). Since the total number of strata is, therefore, the product of the number of subgroups in each factor, the number of strata increases rapidly as factors are added and the levels within factors are refined. Consequently, only the most important variables should be chosen and the number kept to a minimum.

Within each stratum, the randomisation process itself could be simple randomisation, but in practice most clinical trials will use some blocked randomisation approach. As an example, suppose that an investigator wishes to stratify on age and sex, and to use a block size of 4. First, age is divided into a number of categories, say 40–49, 50–59 and 60–69. The design thus has 3 × 2 strata, and the randomisation might be:

Strata	Age	Sex	Group Assignment
1	40–49	Male	ABBA BABA ...
2	40–49	Female	
3	50–59	Male	
4	50–59	Female	
5	60–69	Male	
6	60–69	Female	

Patients between 40–49 years-old and male, would be assigned to treatment groups A and B in the sequences ABBA BABA .... . Similarly random sequences would appear in the other strata.

Although the main argument for stratified randomisation is that of making the treatment groups comparable with respect to specific prognostic factors, it may also lead to increased *power* (see Section 2.3) if the stratification is taken into account in the analysis, by reducing variability in group comparisons. Such reduction allows a study of a given size to detect smaller group differences in outcome measures, or to detect a specified difference with fewer subjects.

Stratified randomisation is of most relevance in small trials, but even here it may not be profitable if there is uncertainty over the importance or reliability of prognostic factors, or if the trial has a limited organisation that might not cope well with complex randomisation procedures. In many cases it may be more useful to employ a *stratified analysis* or analysis of covariance, to adjust for prognostic factors when treament differences are assessed (see later chapters).

2.2.4. Minimisation Method

A further approach to achieving balance between treatment groups on selected prognostic factors is to use an *adaptive randomisation procedure* in which the chance of allocating a new patient to a particular treatment is adjusted according to any existing imbalances in the baseline characteristics of the groups. For example, if sex is a prognostic factor and one treatment group has more women than men, the allocation scheme is such that the next few male patients are more likely to be randomised into the group that currently has fewer men. This method is often referred to as *minimisation*, because imbalances in the distribution of prognostic factors are minimised according to some criterion.

In general, the method is applied in situations involving several prognostic factors and patient allocation is then based on the aim of balancing the marginal treatment totals for each level of each factor.

Table 2.3. Treatment Assignments by Four Prognostic Factors for 80 Patients in a Breast Cancer Trial.

Factor	Level	A	B
Performance status	Ambulatory	30	31
	Non-ambulatory	10	9
Age	< 50	18	17
	≥ 50	22	23
Disease-free interval	< 2 years	31	32
	≥ 2 years	9	8
Dominant metastatic lesion	Visceral	19	21
	Osseous	8	7
	Soft tissue	13	12

(Taken with permission from Pocock, 1983.)

The following example, taken from Pocock (1983), illustrates the procedure:

Table 2.3 shows the number of patients on each of two treatments, A and B, according to each of four prognostic factors. Suppose the next patient is ambulatory, age < 50, has disease-free interval ≥ 2 years and visceral metastasis. Then for each treatment, the number of patients in the corresponding four rows of the table are added:

$$\text{sum for A} = 30 + 18 + 9 + 19 = 76$$

$$\text{sum for B} = 31 + 17 + 8 + 21 = 77$$

Minimisation requires the patient be given the treatment with the smallest marginal total, in this case treatment A. If the sums for A and B were equal, then simple randomisation would be used to assign the treatment.

2.2.5. Unequal Randomisation

Equal-sized treatment groups provide the most efficient means of treatment comparison for any type of outcome measure, and the methods of randomisation described in the previous sections are aimed at achieving what is, in most circumstances, this desirable feature of a trial. (In addition, ideally, each centre in a multi-centre trial should contribute the same number of patients.) But despite the obvious statistical advantages of groups of equal size, there may be other considerations which might require more patients in one group than another. If, for example, the trial is comparing a new treatment against a standard, the investigator might be far more interested in obtaining information about the general charac-teristics of the new treatment, for example, variation in response with dose, than for the old, where such characteristics are likely to be well known. (This is often the situation in early Phase II trials, for which there exist historical data on the standard treatment.) Such infor-mation might be best gained by use of an *unbalanced design* which involves allocating a larger number of patients to the new treatment

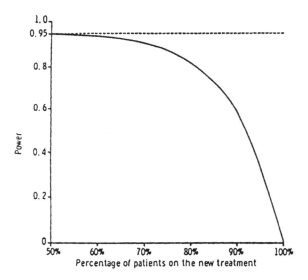

Fig. 2.1. Reduction in power of a trial as the proportion on the new treat-ment is increased (taken with permission from Pocock, 1983).

than to the old. Pocock (1996) gives an example of this approach in a trial for the treatment of advanced breast cancer.

The loss of statistical efficiency in unequal randomisation is considered by Pocock (1983), who shows that if the overall size of a trial is kept constant, its power decreases relatively slowly in the move away from equalsized groups. Figure 2.1 (taken from Pocock, 1983) demonstrates, for example, that power decreases from only 0.95 to 0.925 if 67% of patients are allocated to the new treatment.

The more complex the design, the more difficult it becomes to maintain the integrity of the randomisation process; it becomes vulnerable to both accidental and deliberate misallocation. Consequently, there is much to be said for removing the randomisation decision away from the point of clinical contact, for example, through the use of specialised 24-hour telephone randomisation schemes.

2.3.   THE SIZE OF A CLINICAL TRIAL

According to Simon (1991)

An effective clinical trial must ask an important question and provide a reliable answer. A major determinant of the reliability of the answer is the sample size of the trial. Trials of inadequate size may cause contradictory and erroneous results and thereby lead to an inappropriate treatment of patients. They also divert limited resources from useful applications and cheat the patients who participated in what they thought was important clinical research. Sample size planning is, therefore, a key component of clinical trial methodology.

But, in the recent past at least, such advice has often not been heeded and the literature is dotted with accounts of inconsequential trials. Freiman *et al.* (1978), for example, reviewed 71 'negative' randomised clinical trials, i.e., trials in which the observed differences between the proposed and control treatments were not large enough to satisfy a specified 'significance' level (the risk of a type I error), and the results were declared to be 'not statistically significant'. Analysis of these clinical studies indicated that the investigators often worked with numbers of enrolled patients too small to offer a reasonable chance of avoiding the opposing mistake, a type II error. Fifty of the trials had a greater than 10% risk of missing a substantial difference (true treatment difference of 50%) in the treatment outcome. The reviewers warned that many treatments labelled as 'no different from control' had not received a critical test, because the trials had insufficient power to do the job intended. Such trials are, in a very real sense, unethical in that they require patients to accept the risks of treatment, however small, without any chance of benefit to them or future patients. Small-scale preliminary investigations may be justified when part of a larger plan, but not as an end in their own right (although see later comments).

A specific example of this problem is given by Andersen (1990), who reports a study from the *New England Journal of Medicine*, in which 52 patients with severe cirrhosis and variceal haemorrhage requiring six or more pints of blood were randomly assigned either to sclerotherapy or potocaval shunt. There was no difference in short term survival, with 13 patients in the sclerotherapy group discharged alive, as compared with ten patients in the shunt group. The authors commented as follows:

> We failed to demonstrate any significant difference in long-term survival ... endoscopic sclerotherapy is at least as good as, and may well be better than, definitive early surgical shunting.

The absence of any significant difference made the investigator conclude that one treatment is at least as effective as the other. They failed, however, to consider the possibility of an error of the second kind. A trial with only 26 patients in each group has only a 50–50 chance of a significant result if the true survival rate on one treatment is 25% and on the other twice as much. Even though more patients were discharged alive after sclerotherapy than after portocaval shunt in this study, there remains the distinct possibility that the operation might eventually turn out to be superior.

The deficiency in patient numbers in many clinical trials is, according to Pocock (1996) 'a general phenomena whose full implications for restricting therapeutic progress are not widely appreciated'. In the same article Pocock continues:

The fact is that trials with truly modest treatment effects will achieve statistical significance only if random variation conveniently exaggerated these effects. The chances of publication and reader interest are much greater if the results of the trial are statistically significant. Hence the current obsession with significance testing combined with the inadequate size of many trials means that publications on clinical trials for many treatments are likely to be biased towards as exaggeration of therapeutic effect, even if the trials are unbiased in all other respects.

The combination of high type II error rate, publication bias and the fact that most true treatment advantages are likely to be modest or nonexistent, almost certainly results in a high proportion of false positives in the medical literature, a point also made in Peto *et al.* (1976) and Zelen (1983). Certainly the case against trials with inadequate numbers of subjects appears strong but perhaps with the growing use of *meta-analysis*, a topic to be discussed in Chapter 10, not as strong as is implied by the previous comments.

So how, in designing a trial, is its size arrived at? Although practical and ethical issues need to be considered, most determinations of sample size for a clinical trial are performed, intially at least, in the more statistical context of the hypothesis testing framework of Neyman and Pearson. A null hypothesis is tested at significance level α and the sample size is determined to provide power $1 - \beta$ for rejecting the null when a specified alternative hypothesis is true, where β is the risk of a type II error, i.e., accepting the null hypothesis when it is false. In simple situations the power is a function of three factors:

- the significance level adopted,
- the reliability and variability of the sample data,
- the size of the treatment effect.

The required sample size will be larger the higher the level of significance chosen, the lower the reliability and the smaller the treatment difference hypothesised under the alternative hypothesis. In many trials, the power calculation will also need to include consideration of other factors such as the follow-up time versus number of cases and the number of measurement points.

In this paradigm, the general approach is for the investigator to specify the size of the treatment difference considered clinically relevant (i.e., important to detect) and with what degree of certainty, i.e., with what power, it should be detected. Given such information, the calculation of the corresponding sample size is often relatively straightforward, although the details will depend on the type of response variable and the type of test involved. The last decade has produced a large volume of methodology useful in planning the size of randomised clinical trials with a variety of different types of outcome measures — some examples are to be found in Lee (1983), McHugh and Lee (1984), Schoenfield (1983), Sieh (1987), Wittes and Wallenstein (1987) and Spiegelhalter *et al.* (1994). In many cases, tables are available which enable the required sample size to be simply read off. Increasingly, these are being replaced by computer software for determining sample size for many standard and non-standard designs and outcome measures (see the Appendix).

An obvious danger with such a procedure is that investigators (and, in some cases, their statisticians) may occasionally be led to specify an alternative hypothesis that is unrealistically extreme so that the required sample size looks feasible in terms of possible pressing temporal and financial constraints. Such a possibility may be what led Senn (1997) to describe power calculations as 'a guess masquerading as mathematics' and Pocock (1996) to comment that they are 'a game that can produce any number you wish with manipulative juggling of the parameter values'. Statisticians advising on clinical trials need to be active in estimating the degree of difference that can be realistically expected for a clinical trial based on previous studies of a particular disease or, when such information is lacking, perhaps based on subjective opinions of investigators and physicians *not* involved in the proposed trial.

2.4. REPORTING RESULTS

The first part of a trial report should be descriptive and summarise the patient pool, the study protocol and the characteristics of those entered. Appropriate graphical material should be included here. Following this will be the results of the various statistical analyses performed. In many cases the analyses will involve the application of one or other significance test and what is often tabulated is the p-value associated with the test. Unfortunately and despite the many caveats in the literature, the accept/reject philosophy of significance testing remains dominant in the minds of many non-statisticians, who appear determined to continue to experience joy on finding a p-value of 0.049 and despair on finding one of only 0.051. A decade ago, Gardner and Altman (1986) made the point that the excessive use of hypothesis testing at the expense of other ways of assessing results had reached such a degree that levels of significance were often quoted alone in the main text and abstracts of papers, with no mention of actual concentrations, proportions, etc., or their differences. The implications of hypothesis testing — that there can always be a simple 'yes' or 'no' answer as the fundamental result from a medical study — is clearly false, and used in this way hypothesis testing is of limited value.

So should statisticians be encouraging the abandonment of the p-value altogether? Many statisticians might be tempted to answer 'yes', but a more sensible response is perhaps a resounding 'maybe'. Such values should rarely be used in a purely confirmatory way, but in an exploratory fashion they can give some informal guidance on the possible existence of an interesting effect, even when the required assumptions of whatever test is being used are known to be only partially valid. It is often possible to assess whether a p-value is likely to be an under- or overestimate, and whether the result is clear one way or the other.

Fortunately, the use of significance testing appears to have become less obsessive and dogmatic during the last few years, with greater emphasis on statistical estimation and confidence intervals. The latter, which can be considered to be the set of true but unknown differences that are statistically compatible with the observed difference, can be found relatively simply for many quantities of interest (see Gardner and Altman, 1986), and although the underlying logic of interval estimates is essentially similar to that of significance tests, they do not carry with them the pseudo scientific decision making language of such tests. Instead they give a plausible range of values for the unknown parameter, with, for example, inadequate sample size being signalled by the sheer width of the interval. As Oakes (1986) rightly comments:

> The significance test relates to what a population parameter is *not*: the confidence interval gives a plausible range for what the parameter *is*.

Since clinical trials are generally designed to provide *global* treatment comparisons, which may not be suited to the needs of individual patients, a question which frequently arises when reporting results, whether as p-values or confidence intervals, is how to identify particular subgroups of patients who responded well (or badly) to a new treatment? Answering such a question is relatively easy — such *subgroup analysis* can be carried out using standard statistical techniques such as analysis of variance or the like. If, for example, subgroups were formed on the basis of sex (male, female) and age (young, old), then with a two treatment trial, a $2 \times 2 \times 2$ ANOVA on the response variable of interest could be performed and all possible interactions and main effects assessed in the usual way. But many statisticians would recommend that such analyses are better avoided altogether, or if undertaken, interpreted extremely cautiously in the spirit of 'exploration' rather than anything more formal. Their reasons are not difficult to identify:

- trials can rarely provide sufficient power to detect such subgroup effects,
- there are often many possible prognostic factors from which to form subgroups, so that the analysis may degenerate into 'data dredging',
- the temptation to over interpret an apparent subgroup finding is likely to be difficult to resist (Yusuf *et al.*, 1991).

Chapter 10 (Fig. 10.2 and Table 10.1) provides a checklist for what is currently expected that studies should report.

2.5. SUMMARY

In this chapter three aspects of the design of clinical trials has been considered: the allocation of patients to treatments, the size of the trial, and how to report results. The well documented chaos that can result from non-randomised trials has led to a general acceptance of randomisation as an essential component of the vast majority of trials. Several methods of randomisation have been considered in this chapter, but there are others that have not been mentioned, in particular *cluster randomisation* in which natural groupings of individuals, for example, general practices, become the units of randomisation, and *play the winner rules*, in which the randomisation is biased to allow a higher proportion of future allocations to the treatment with (currently) better observed outcome. The former are described in Donner and Klar (1994) and are increasingly important in, for example, country intervention trials. The latter presumably arise from the desire amongst some clinicians for more 'ethically acceptable' allocation procedures, but there have been very few clinical trials that have actually used such data-dependent procedures. Pocock

(1996) points to both the impracticality of implementation (early results usually arrive too late) and the suspicions of bias in allocations (the result, for example, of secular trends in the type of patient recruited) as reasons that such approaches continue to be largely regarded as 'statistical curiosities' rather than serious contenders for clinical applications.

Statisticians have been very effective in developing methodology for determining sample size in randomised clinical trials. Nevertheless, there is continuing evidence that many reported trials are too small, leading to a high type II error rate as well as a low proportion of true positive to false positive findings. Meta-analysis (see Chapter 10) may help with this problem, but it is unlikely to provide a completely satisfactory answer in all cases.

Ten years ago the results of most clinical trials were given in terms of p-values. The situation has now changed for the better, with many medical journals rightly demanding confidence intervals. The problem with significance testing would not be so bad if only a single test (or a very small number) was carried out per trial. Most trials, however, generate large amounts of data and dozens of significance tests from the results of using such procedures as *interim analyses* and employing *multiple endpoints*, topics to be discussed in the next two chapters.

CHAPTER 3

Monitoring Trial Progress: Outcome Measures, Compliance, Dropouts and Interim Analyses

3.1. INTRODUCTION

The basic elements of the plan for any trial will be set long before the first patient is enrolled, and will, eventually, be translated into the study protocol. Here the primary objectives of the trial will be detailed in terms of type of patients to be studied, class of treatments to be evaluated and primary outcome measures. In addition, the document will specify the number of patients to be recruited (usually from the results of a sample size calculation), required length of patient follow-up, patient entry and exclusion criteria, method of randomisation, details of pre-randomisation procedures and other general organisational structures.

Putting the study plan into execution begins with patient recruitment, a period which is crucial in the life of a trial, although the details need not delay us here, since the various possible problems and pitfalls are well documented in, for example, Meinert (1986).

Once a trial has started, various aspects of a patient's progress need to be assessed. Investigators are, for example, under a strict obligation to report unexpected adverse events as they occur since these may necessitate withdrawing of a patient from the trial.

The problem of patient compliance must also be addressed. The optimal study from a compliance point of view is one in which the investigator has total control over the patient, the administration of the intervention regimen and follow-up. But in practice, there is very likely to be less than 100% compliance with the intervention and clearly the results of a trial can be affected by noncompliance; it can, for example, lead to an underreporting of possible therapeutic as well as toxic effects. This has the potential to undermine even a properly designed trial and consequently, monitoring compliance is generally critical in a clinical trial, a point taken up in detail in Section 3.3.

A patient's performance during a clinical trial is characterised by measurements on one or more outcome variables. These measurements need to be made in as objective, accurate and consistent a manner as possible and in a way that should be precisely defined in the study protocol, issues that are discussed more fully in Section 3.2.

In most clinical trials, patients are entered one at a time so that their responses to treatment are also observed sequentially. The accumulating data in a trial needs to be monitored for a variety of reasons. In addition to checking for compliance and noting possible adverse side effects, monitoring is also needed to assess whether early termination of the trial might be necessary. Early termination might be called for if there was an indication that the intervention was harmful to patients. Alternatively, if the data indicate a clear benefit from the intervention, the trial may need to be stopped early because to continue to use the control treatment would be unethical. The handling of treatment comparisons while a trial is still in progress poses some difficult statistical problems which are taken up in Section 3.4.

3.2. OUTCOME MEASURES

The outcome measure(s) used for treatment comparisons may be a clinical event, for example, death or recurrence of a disease, or a measurement of some other characteristics of interest, for example, blood pressure, serum lipid level or breathing difficulties. Such observations and measurements are the raw material of the trial and they clearly need to be objective, precise and reproducible for reasons nicely summarised by the following quotation from Fleiss (1986):

> The most elegant design of a clinical study will not overcome the damage caused by unreliable or imprecise measurement. The requirement that one's data be of high quality is at least as important a component of a proper study design as the requirement for randomisation, double blinding, controlling where necessary for prognostic factors and so on. Larger sample sizes than otherwise necessary, biased estimates, and even biased samples are some of the untoward consequences of unreliable measurements that can be demonstrated.

So no trial is better than the quality of its data and quality control begins with clear definitions of response variables. The decision about which, when and how measurements are to be made needs to be taken *before* the trial commences. The alternative is potential chaos. Attention clearly needs to be given to training clinicians and others on the measuring instruments to be used; this is particularly important in multi-centre trials. Results from studies based on poorly standardised procedures that use ambiguous definitions or conducted by insufficiently trained staff, can lead to both loss of power and bias in the estimate of treatment effect. Most properly conducted trials will, in fact, have well developed systems in place for data quality control and auditing. The purpose of such a system is to provide reasonable assurance to the organisers of the trial as well as to the 'consumers' of the results that the data on which the conclusions are based are reliable. Some practical issues in assuring such quality control of the data generated in clinical trials are discussed in Knatterud *et al.* (1998).

The measurements made in many trials will involve rating scales of one type or another, for example, quality-of-life assessments. When there has been little experience of using such scales or where they have only been recently developed, it may be important to investigate their *reliability*, i.e., the extent to which measurements of the same subject made by different observers agree. In most trials, particularly multi-centre trials, the problem of observer variation will need to be confronted. A formal assessment of the reliability of the instrument to be used may even be necessary. Readers are referred to the comprehensive accounts of assessing reliability in both Fleiss (1986) and Dunn (1989) for details.

In some trials the outcome measure of substantive interest may not be measured for practical and/or ethical reasons. Instead a *surrogate* variable is selected on which to investigate treatment differences. If, for example, we measure blood pressure rather than say the potential problems of high blood pressure, we are using a surrogate measure. Other examples include bone mineral density in the treatment of osteoporosis rather than the rate of bone fracture, and CD4 counts rather than deaths in the treatment of AIDS.

The aim in using such surrogate measures is to assess the treatment effect with less trouble and perhaps greater efficiency than by using the preferred endpoint. But the dangers of not using the true endpoint cannot be dismissed lightly. Senn (1997) points out that the demonstration of a high correlation between the proposed surrogate measure and the measure of substantive interest does not ensure that using the former will be adequate. He uses the treatment of oestoporosis measured by bone mineral density (BMD) as an example. Loss of BMD leads to a weakening of bones and an increased risk of fracture. If, however, a treatment increases density but at the expense of adversely affecting the construction of the bones it may actually have a harmful effect on the fracture rate. The implication is that the adequacy of a surrogate measure may depend on the treatment, a possibility recognised by the USA drugs regulatory body, the *Food and Drug Administration* (FDA) guidelines for oesteoporosis studies, these requiring the measure of fractures for bisphophonates but accepting BMD for hormone replacement.

3.3. COMPLIANCE, DROPOUTS AND INTENTION-TO-TREAT

There could be no worse experimental animals on earth than human beings; they complain, they go on vacations, they take things they are not supposed to take, they lead incredibly complicated lives, and, sometimes, they do not take their medicine. (Efron, 1998.)

Compliance means following both the intervention regimen and trial procedures (for example, clinic visits, laboratory procedures and filling out forms). A non-complier is a patient who fails to meet the standards of compliance as established by the investigator. A high degree of patient compliance is an important aspect of a well-run trial.

But treatment compliance is rarely an all-or-none phenomena. The level of compliance achieved may range from low to high, depending on both the patient and the staff. Perfect compliance is probably impossible to achieve, particularly in drug trials where the patient maybe required to take the assigned medication at the same time of day over long periods of time. Lack of compliance can take a number of forms; the patient can drop out of the trial, take none of the medication (whilst perhaps pretending to do so), forget to take the treatment from time to time, or take it at the wrong time, etc.

Level of compliance will depend on a number of factors, including:

- The amount of time and inconvenience involved in making follow-up visits to the clinic,
- The perceived importance of the procedures performed at each visit from a health maintenance point of view,
- The potential health benefits associated with treatment versus potential risks,

- The amount of discomfort produced by the study treatments or procedures performed,
- The amount of effort required of the patient to maintain the treatment regime,
- The number and type of side effects associated with treatment.

In recent times the problems of noncompliance in a clinical trial have been well illustrated in trials involving HIV/AIDS patients, where an atmosphere of rapidly alternating hopes and disappointments has added to the difficulties of keeping patients on a fixed long-term treatment schedule.

So what can be done to ensure maximal patient compliance? Aspects of the study design may help; the shorter the trial, for example, the more likely subjects are to comply with the intevention regimen. So a study started and completed in one day would have great advantages over longer trials. And studies in which the subjects are under close supervision, such as in-patient hospital-based trials, tend to have fewer problems of noncompliance.

Simplicity of intervention may also affect compliance, with single dose drug regimens usually being preferable to those requiring multiple doses. The interval between scheduled visits to hospital or clinic is also a factor to consider. Too long an interval between visits may lead to a steady fall in patient compliance due to lack of encouragement, while too short an interval may prove a nuisance and reduce cooperation.

Perhaps the most important factor in maintaining good subject compliance once a trial has begun is the attitude of the staff running the trial. Experienced investigators stay in close contact with the patients early after randomisation to get patients involved and, later, to keep them interested when their initial enthusiasm may have worn off. On the other hand, uninterested or discourteous staff will lead to an uninterested patient population. Meinert (1986) lists a number of simple factors likely to enhance patient participation and interest; this list is reproduced here in Table 3.1.

Table 3.1. Factors and Approaches that Enhance Patient Interest and Participation.

- Clinic staff who treat patients with courtesy and dignity and who take an interest in meeting their needs,
- Clinic located in pleasant physical surroundings and in a secure environment,
- Convenient access to parking for patients who drive, and to other modes of transportation for those who do not,
- Payment of parking and travel fees incurred by study patients,
- Payment of clinic registration fees and costs for procedures required in the trial,
- Special clinics in which patients are able to avoid the confusion and turmoil of a regular out-patient clinic,
- Scheduled appointments designed to minimise waiting time,
- Clinic hours designed for patient convenience,
- Written or telephone contacts between clinic visits,
- Remembering patients on special occasions, such as Christmas, birthday anniversaries, etc.,
- Establishment of identity with the study through proper indoctrination and explanantion of study procedures during the enrollment process; through procedures such as the use of special ID cards to identify the patient as a participant in the study, and by awarding certificates to recognise their contributions to the trial.

(Taken with permission from Meinert, 1986.)

Monitoring compliance is a crucial part of many clinical trials, since according to Freidman, Furberg and DeMets (1985):

... the interpretation of study results will be influenced by knowledge of compliance with the intervention. To the extent that the control group is not truly a control group and the intervention group is not being treated as intended, group differences may be diluted, leading possibly to an underestimate of the therapeutic effect and an underreporting of adverse effects.

Feinstein (1974) points out that differential compliance to two equally effective regimens can also lead to possibly erroneous conclusions about the effect of the intervention.

In some studies measuring compliance is relatively easy. For example, trials in which one group receives surgery and the other group does not. Most of the time, however, assessment of compliance is not so simple and can rarely be established perfectly. In drug trials one of the most commonly used methods of evaluating subject compliance is pill or capsule count. But the method is far from foolproof. Even when a subject returns the appropriate number of leftover pills at a scheduled visit, the question of whether the remaining pills were used according to the protocol remains largely unanswered. Good rapport with the subjects will encourage cooperation and lead to a more accurate pill count, although there is considerable evidence that shows that the method can be unreliable and potentially misleading (see, for example, Cramer *et al.*, 1988, and Waterhouse *et al.*, 1993).

Laboratory determinations can also sometimes be used to monitor compliance to medications. Tests done on either blood or urine can detect the presence of active drugs or metabolites. For example, Hjalmarson *et al.* (1981) checked compliance with metroprobol therapy after myocardial infarction by using assays of metroprobol in urine. Several other approaches to monitoring compliance are described in Freidman, Furberg and Demets (1985), and Senn (1997) mentions two recent technical developments which may be useful, namely:

- Electronic monitoring — pill dispensers with a built-in microchip which will log when the dispenser was opened,
- Low-dose, slow turnover chemical markers which can be added to treatment and then detected via blood-sampling.

The claim is often made that in published drug trials more than 90% of patients have been satisfactorily compliant with the protocol-specified dosing regimen. But Urquhart and DeKlerk (1998) sugest that these claims, based as they usually are, on count of returned dosing forms, which patients can easily manipulate, are exaggerated, and that data from the more reliable methods for measuring compliance mentioned above, contadict them.

Noncompliance may lead to the investigator transferring a patient to the alternative therapy or withdrawing the patient from the study altogether; often such decisions are taken out of the investigators hands by the patient simply refusing to participate in the trial any further and thus becoming a trial *dropout.* When noncompliance manifests as dropout from a study, the connection with missing data is direct (see Section 3.3.2). In other circumstances manifestation of noncompliance is more complex and some response is observed, but a question remains about what would have been observed had compliance been achieved.

Noncompliance, leading either to receiving treatment other than that provided for by the results of randomisation, or to dropping out of the trial altogether, has serious implications for the analysis of the data collected in a clinical trial, implications which will be discussed briefly here and taken up again in later chapters.

3.3.1. Intention-to-Treat

As indicated above, in most randomised clinical trials not all patients adhere to the therapy to which they were randomly assigned. Instead they may receive the therapy assigned to another treatment group, or even a therapy different from any prescribed in the protocol. When such non-adherence occurs, problems arise with the analysis comparing the treatments under study. There are a number of possibilities of which the following are the most common:

- *Intention-to-treat* or *analysis-as-randomised* in which analysis is based on original treatment assignment rather than treatment actually received,
- *Adherers-only method*, i.e., analysing only those patients who adhered to the original treatment assignment,
- *Treatment-received method*, i.e., analysing patients according to the treatment ultimately received.

The intention-to-treat (ITT) approach requires that any comparison of the treatments is based upon comparison of the outcome results of all patients in the treatment groups to which they were randomly assigned. This approach is recommended since it maintains the benefits of randomisation, whereas the second and third of the methods above compare groups that have *not* been randomised to their respective treatments; consequently, the analyses maybe subject to unknown biases and for this reason most statisticians and drug regulatory agencies prefer intention-to-treat. But although it is clear that analyses based on compliance are inherently biased because non-compliance does not occur randomly, many clinicians (and even some statisticians) have criticised analysis that does not reflect the treatment actually received, especially when many patients do not remain on the initially assigned therapy (see, for example, Feinstein, 1991). In the face of substantial non-compliance, it is not difficult to understand the intuitive appeal of comparing only those patients in the original trial that actually complied with the prescribed treatment. However, in addition to the difficulty of defining compliance in an objective manner, subjects who comply tend to fare differently and in a somewhat unpredictable way from those who do not comply. Thus any observed difference among treatment groups constructed in this way may be due not to treatment but to factors associated with compliance.

Dissatisfaction with analysis by original treatment assignment arises because of its apparent failure to evaluate the 'true' effect of the treatment. According to Dixon and Albert (1995), an intention-to-treat analysis determines treatment effectiveness where this involves both compliance on treatment, as well as its biological effect, whereas an as-treated analysis assesses treatment efficacy. This, however, appears to simply be ignoring the potential problem of bias in the latter.

Peduzzi *et al.* (1993) compare the various methods of analysis on data from a randomised trial of coronary artery bypass surgery designed to compare the survival times of patients assigned optimal medical therapy with those assigned coronary bypass surgery.

Amongst the 354 patients assigned to medical therapy, the cumulative 14-year crossover rate from medical to surgical therapy was 55%. In contrast, only 20 of the 332 patients assigned to surgical therapy refused surgery. Analysis by the as-randomised approach indicated that the treatment groups were statistically indistinguishable. In contrast the analyses by adherers-only and by treatment received indicated an apparent consistent survival advantage with surgical therapy throughout the entire 14-year follow-up period, although the advantage begins to diminish with extended follow-up. The authors demonstrate that the apparent survival advantage arises from the striking difference in survival between the crossovers to surgery and the medical adherers.

In the same paper, some simulated data are used to emphasise the problems with other than an as-randomised analysis. One example presented involves simulated data for a hypothetical cohort of 350 medical and 350 surgical patients having exponentially distributed survival times and assuming a 10-year survival rate of 50% in each group. In addition, they generated an independent exponential time to 'crossover' for each of the 350 medical patients assuming half the patients crossed over by 10 years. Medical crossovers were then defined as those patients with time to crossover less than survival time. Figure 3.1 displays 10-year survival rates by the as-randomised, adherers-only, and treatment-received methods. The latter two methods demonstrate a consistent survival advantage in favour of surgical therapy, when by definition here, there is actually no difference in survival between the two treatment groups.

According to Efron (1998), 'Statistics deals with the analysis of complicated noisy phenomena, never more so than in its applications to biomedical research, and in this noisy world the intent-to-treat analysis of a randomised double-blinded clinical trial stands as a flagpole of certainty amongst the chaos.' Indeed, according to Goetghebeur and Shapiro (1993), intention-to-treat analysis has achieved the status of a 'Buick' — 'Best Unbiased Inference with regard to Causal Knowledge'. Many statisticians would endorse these views

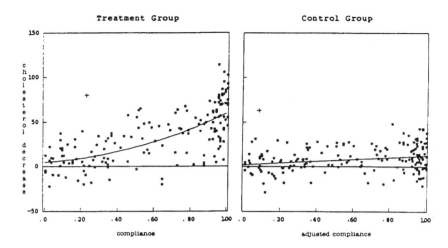

Fig. 3.1. Compliance dose-response curves for decrease in cholesterol level in active treatment and control groups in a trial of cholestyramine (taken with permission from Peduzzi *et al.*, 1993).

and also find themselves largely in agreement with Peduzzi *et al.* (1993):

> We conclude that the method of analysis should be consistent with the experimental design of a study. For randomised trials, such consistency requires the preservation of the random treatment assignment. Because methods that violate the principles of randomisation are susceptible to bias, we are against their use.

But despite widespread agreement amongst statisticians that intention-to-treat analysis remains the most appropriate way to deal with noncompliance, there is growing interest in how to take compliance information into account without fatally compromising the conclusions of a randomised clinical trial, particularly now that measurement of compliance can be made more reliable. (Dunn, 1999, considers the problem of measurement error in assessing compliance.) There have been several attempts to incorporate compliance data into the analysis of clinical trials and to devise analytic methods

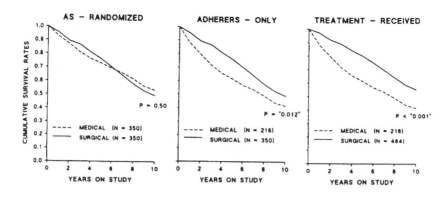

Fig. 3.2. Ten-year survival rates by the as-randomised, adherers-only and treatment-received approaches for a set of simulated data (taken with permission from Efron and Feldman, 1991).

that adjust for noncompliance. Examples include Efron and Feldman (1991), Pocock and Abdalla (1998), and Robins (1998). Efron and Feldman, for example, discuss a trial concerned with the effectiveness of the drug cholestyramine for lowering cholesterol levels, in which each patient's compliance was assessed by the proportion of the intended dose actually taken. Figure 3.2 shows the relationship between compliance and the decrease in cholesterol level for both treatment and control groups. A 'dose-response' relation is evident for *both* groups; better compliance leads to a greater decrease in cholesterol level, as indicated by the quadratic regression curves. But the curves shown are *compliance* dose-response curves; they may not give an accurate picture of the true dose-response curve because compliance (and hence dose) has not been assigned in a randomised fashion by the investigators. Compliance is an uncontrolled covariate, and it may be that better compliers are better patients to begin with. This seems very likely given the nature of the observed curve in the control group. Efron and Feldman describe how the true dose-response curve can be recovered from the treatment and control compliance-response curves.

Pocock and Abdalla (1998), whilst accepting that analysis by intention-to-treat remains the statistical approach for presenting the comparative results of different treatment policies within a randomised controlled trial, comment on the growing interest in exploring more complex statistical approaches which incorporate measures of individual patient compliance with the intended treatment regimens into supplementary comparative analyses. They offer an example from their own analysis of a three-arm study of cardiology patients, testing a beta-blocker and a diuretic versus placebo. As expected, the diuretic group showed a tendency to increased serum cholesterol levels, but unexpectedly the same effect showed up in the beta-blocker group. It was discovered, however, that 30% of the beta-blocker group was also taking diuretics, and the beta-blocker cholesterol effect disappeared when this fact was incorporated in the analysis.

In the past the inclusion of compliance measurements in the analysis of clinical trials has been fiercely resisted by many statisticians, and if not resisted, largely ignored. But in Efron's view (Efron, 1998), this will change and at some time in the not too distant future, it will seem as wrong to run a clinical trial without compliance measurement as without randomisation. The statistical challenge, according to Sir David Cox (Cox, 1998), will be to develop methods of analysis that take account of the complex character of compliance without analyses becoming too complicated conceptually. He warns of the dangers of treating compliance as a simple binary, yes, no, concept and also of ignoring the nature and the essential reason for noncompliance since this may vary greatly between individuals.

The most extreme form of noncompliance occurs when patients drop-out of a trial prematurely. Dealing with dropouts can present challenging problems in analysing the results from the trial. The next section presents a taxonomy of dropouts which will be of importance in later analysis chapters.

3.3.2.   A Taxonomy of Dropouts

The design of most clinical trials specifies that all patients are to have the measurement of the outcome variable(s) made at a common set

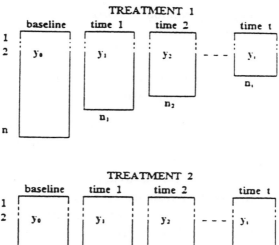

Fig. 3.3. Monotone data pattern caused by patients dropping out of trial.

of time points leading to what might be termed a *balanced* data set. But although balanced longitudinal data is generally the aim, *unbalanced* data is often what the investigator is faced with because of the occurrence of *missing values* in the sense that intended measurements are not taken, are lost, or are otherwise unavailable. Staff, for example, may fail to make a scheduled observation, or patients may miss an appointment. This type of missing value usually occurs intermittently. In contrast, dropping out of a clinical trial implies that once an observation at a particular time point is missing so are all subsequent planned observations, giving rise to a *monotone* data pattern (see Fig. 3.3).

Assumptions about the probability model for missing data can influence both the analysis and interpretation of the longitudinal data collected in clinical trials. In the statistical literature three types of dropout have been distinguished:

- Missing completely random (MCAR),
- Missing at random (MAR),
- Non-ignorable (sometimes referred to as informative).

To explain the distinction between these three types it is necessary to introduce a little nomenclature:

- For each patient it is planned to make a sequence of T observations, $Y_1, Y_2, \ldots, Y_T$. In addition for each patient, there may be a set of fixed covariates, X, assumed fully observed.
- Missing values arise from individuals dropping out, so that if Y_k is missing, then so also are $Y_{k+1}, \ldots, Y_T$.
- Define a dropout indicator D for each patient, where $D = k$ if the patient drops out between the $(k-1)$th and kth observation time, and $D = T + 1$ if the patient does not drop out.

Completely random dropout (MCAR) occurs when patients dropout of the study in a process which is independent of both the observed measurements and those that would have been available had they not been missing, so that

$$P(D = k|X, Y_1, Y_2, \ldots, Y_T) = P(D = k)$$

Here the observed (nonmissing) values effectively constitue a simple random sample of the values for all study subjects. Examples of MCAR dropout might be data missing due to accidental death or because a patient has moved to another district. Intermittent missing values in a longitudinal data set might also be assumed to be MCAR, though supporting evidence would usually be required. Completely random dropout causes least problems for data analyses.

Additionally, data may be missing due to design, but still be independent of the outcome values. An example would be a study designed to have less frequent assessments in a group having a standard treatment. Little (1995), distinguishes completely random drop-out from *covariate-dependent* dropout, for which

$$\Pr(D = k|X, Y_1, \ldots, Y_T) = \Pr(D = k|X)$$

and the probability of dropping out depends on the values of the fixed covariates X, but given X, it is conditionally independent of an individual's outcome values, $Y_1, \ldots, Y_T$. Such a definition allows dependence of drop-out on both between-subject and within-subject covariates that can be treated as fixed in the model. In particular, if X includes treatment-group indicators, this definition allows the dropout rates to vary over treatment groups and seasonal dropout effects could be modelled by including season indicators as within-subject covariates in the model.

Random dropout (MAR) occurs when the dropout process depends on the outcome measures that have been observed in the past, but given this information is conditionally independent of all the future (unrecorded) values of the outcome variable following dropout, so that

$$P(D = k|X, Y_1, \ldots, Y_T) = P(D = k|X, Y_1, \ldots, Y_{k-1})$$

Here 'missingness' depends only on the observed data with the distribution of future values for a subject who drops out at time t being the same as the distribution of the future values of a subject who remains in at time t, if they have the same covariates and the same past history of outcome up to and including time t. An example of a set of data in which the dropouts violate the MCAR assumption but *may* be MAR is shown in Fig. 3.4, taken from Curran *et al.* (1998). The diagram shows mean physical functioning scores by time of dropout; higher scores represent a higher level of functioning. We can see that patients with a lower physical functioning tended to dropout of the study earlier than patients with a higher physical functioning score. Consequently, the probability of dropout depended on the previous functioning score and hence the dropout was not MCAR.

Finally, in the case of non-ignorable or informative dropout, the dropout process, $P(D = k|X, Y_1, \ldots, Y_T)$ depends on the unobserved values of the outcome variable. That is, dropout is said to be non-ignorable when the probability of dropout depends on the unrecorded values of the outcome variable that would have been observed had

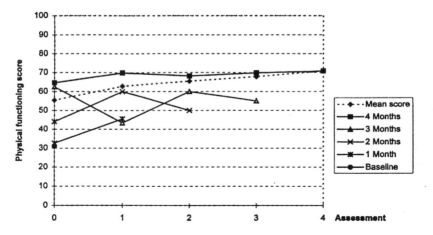

Fig. 3.4. Physical functioning score by time of dropout (taken with permission from Curran *et al.*, 1998).

the patient remained in the study. An example given by Cnaan, Laird and Slasor (1997) involves trials of patients undergoing chemotherapy treatment for cancer, in which quality-of-life assessments are required on a quarterly basis. Most quality-of-life forms are self-report and may require substantial effort on the part of the patient. Patients who are experiencing poor quality-of-life are likely to be far less able to complete the self-report required for response. In this case obtaining valid estimates of population parameters is likely to be far more complicated since we are in a situation of having to make assumptions about the distribution of missing values which cannot be fully tested by the data.

The full implications of this taxonomy of dropouts for the analysis of longitudinal data from clinical trials will be made explicit in later chapters.

3.4. INTERIM ANALYSES IN CLINICAL TRIALS

The Tuskegee Syphillis Study was initiated in the USA in 1932 and continued into the early 1970s. The study involved enrollment and follow-up of 400 untreated latent syphilitic black males (and 200 un-infected controls) in order to trace the course of the disease. In recent years, the trial has come under severe criticism because of the fact that the syphilitics remained untreated even when penicillin, an accepted form of treatment for the disease, became available. Ma-jor ethical questions arise if investigators elect to continue a medical experiment beyond the point at which the evidence in favour of an effective treatment is unequivocal.

Clearly then, it is ethically desirable to terminate a clinical trial earlier than originally planned if one therapy is clearly shown to be superior than the alternatives under test. (This may apply even if it is a *different* concurrent study which reports such a result.) But as mentioned in the Introduction to this chapter, in most clin-ical trials patients are entered one at a time and their responses to treatment observed sequentially. Assessing these accumulating data for evidence of a treatment difference large and convincing enough to terminate the trial is rarely straightforward. Indeed the decision to stop accrual to a clinical trial early is often difficult and multifaceted. The procedure most widely adopted is a *planned* series of *interim analyses* to be done at a limited number of pre-specified points during the course of the trial. Because the data are examined after groups of observations rather than after each observation, the name *group sequential* is often used. A number of such methods have been proposed, some of which will be discussed in more detail later in this section. The aim of all the different approaches, however, is to overcome the potential problems that can arise from repeated tests of significance or *multiple testing*.

The problem of taking 'multiple looks' at the accumulating data in a clinical trial has been addressed by many authors including Anscombe (1954), Armitage *et al.* (1969), McPherson (1982), Pocock (1982) and O'Brien and Fleming (1979). The problem is that, if on each 'look' the investigator follows conventional rules for interpreting the resulting p-value, then *inappropriate* rejection of the null hypoth-esis of no treatment difference will occur too often. In other words,

Table 3.2. Repeated Significance Tests on Accumulating Data.

Number of Repeated Tests at the 5% Level	Overall Significance Level
1	0.05
2	0.08
3	0.11
4	0.13
5	0.14
10	0.19
20	0.25
50	0.32
100	0.37
1000	0.53
∞	1.0

(Taken with permission from Pocock, 1983.)

repeatedly testing interim data can inflate false positive rates if not handled appropriately. Armitage *et al.* (1969) give the actual significance levels corresponding to various numbers of interim analyses for a normally distributed test statistic; these values are shown in Table 3.2. So, for example, if five interim analyses are performed, the chance of at least one showing a treatment difference at the 5% level, when the null hypothesis is true, is 0.14. As Cornfield (1976) comments:

Just as the Sphinx winks if you look at it too long, so, if you perform enough significance tests, you are sure to find significance even when none exists.

An example of this problem described by Freidman, Furberg and DeMets (1985) involved a trial comparing mortality in clofibrate and placebo treated patients in the Coronary Drug Project (1981). In the

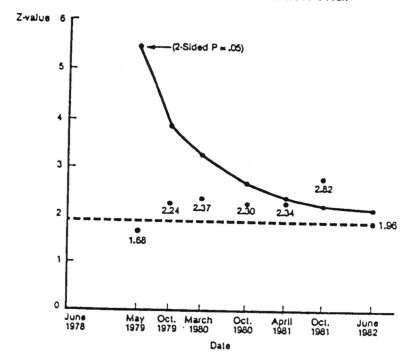

Fig. 3.5. Results from a trial comparing mortality in clofibrate and placebo treated patients (taken with permission from Freidman, Furberg and DeMets, 1985).

early months of the study, clofibrate appeared to be beneficial, with the significance level exceeding 5% on three occasions (see Fig. 3.5). However, because of the repeated testing issue, the decision was made to continue the study and closely monitor the results. The early difference was not maintained, and at the end of the trial the drug showed no benefit over placebo. Such a difference might arise for a variety of reasons, including:

- early patients in a trial are not always representative of the later patients,

- number of events are small,
- randomisation may not yet have achieved balance.

The basic strategy involved in the group sequential approach is to define a critical value at each interim analysis $(Z_c(k), k = 1, \ldots, K)$ such that the overall type I error rate will be maintained at a prespecified level. At each interim analysis, the accumulating standardised test statistic $(Z(k), k = 1, \ldots, K)$ is compared to the critical value where K is the maximum number of interim analyses planned for. The trial is continued if the magnitude of the test statistic is less than the critical value, for that interim analysis. Various sequences of critical values have been proposed. Pocock (1977), for example, suggested that the critical value should be constant for all analyses. But O'Brien and Fleming (1979) proposed changing critical values over the K interim analyses. Peto *et al.* (1976) suggested that a large critical value be used for each interim analysis and then for the last analysis, the usual critical value should be utilised. Example of the Pocock, O'Brien and Fleming, and Peto *et al.* boundaries for $K = 5$ and $\alpha = 0.05$ (two-sided) are shown in Fig. 3.6. (A brief account of the type of calculation behind these boundaries is given later.)

For each of the approaches mentioned above the number of interim analyses, K, has to be specified in advance, but Lan and DeMets (1983) consider a more general method (the *alpha spending procedure*) to implement group sequential boundaries that control the type I error rate while allowing flexibility in how many interim analyses are to be conducted and at what times.

Pampallona and Tsiatis (1994) introduce a class of boundaries for group sequential clinical trials that allow for early stopping when small treatment differences are observed. The boundaries can be derived exactly for any choice of type I and type II error probabilities, and can be easily applied to both one- and two-sided hypothesis testing. A brief account of how these boundaries are derived is given in Table 3.3, while Table 3.4 (adapted from Pampallona and Tsiatis, 1994) gives values of the boundaries for various combinations of the design parameters. In general, however, the boundaries required for

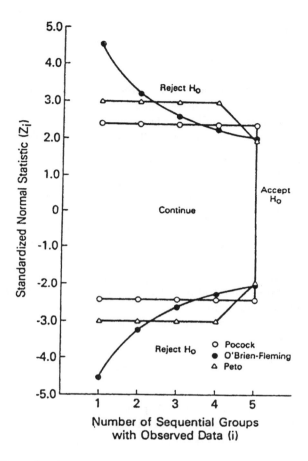

Fig. 3.6. Pocock, O'Brien and Fleming and Peto *et al.* boundaries for interim analyses (taken with permission from Lan and DeMets, 1983).

most proposed group sequential procedures are most easily obtained using the specialised software described in the Appendix. As an illustration, we will consider an example from the EaSt manual (see the Appendix) which involves a trial comparing a new compound with a standard treatment for the control of systolic blood pressure. The expectation is that systolic blood pressure should decrease to about 95 mmHg with the new drug, against the current 105 mmHg

Table 3.3. Obtaining Boundaries for Group Sequential Analysis.

- The problem is one of comparing the effectiveness of two treatments, A and B say.
- Let the response be normally distributed with expected values μ_A and μ_B respectively, and common variance σ^2.
- It is required to test the null hypothesis of treatment equivalence, namely $H_0 : \mu_A = \mu_B = \delta = 0$, against the alternative hypothesis, $H_1 : \delta \neq 0$.
- Patients will enter the randomised trial in a staggered fashion over time and the accumulating responses are analysed each time an additional group of n observations become available on each treatment arm, with the goal of interrupting accrual into the trial whenever a large treatment difference is observed.
- Let the maximum number of planned analyses be K, so that the maximum sample size should the trial be required to continue until the last analysis, is $N = 2Kn$ patients.
- The testing strategy consists of stopping the study, and either accepting H_0 or H_1, the first time the test statistic takes a value outside a suitably defined continuation region.
- The test statistic at the jth analysis is defined as:

$$S_j = \sum_{i=1}^{j} \frac{\sum_{l=1}^{n} x_{ilA} - \sum_{l=1}^{n} x_{ilB}}{\sigma\sqrt{2n}}$$

  where x_{ilA} and x_{ilB} denote the responses of the lth patient in the ith group on treatment A and B, respectively.
- The statistic S_j is a partial sum of normal random variables, Y_i, of the form:

$$Y_i \frac{\sum_{l=1}^{n} x_{ilA} - \sum_{l=1}^{n} x_{ilB}}{\sigma\sqrt{2n}} \sim N(\delta^*, 1)$$

  where

$$\delta^* = \frac{(\mu_A - \mu_B)\sqrt{n}}{\sigma\sqrt{2}} = \frac{\delta\sqrt{n}}{\sigma\sqrt{2}}$$

- The group sequential approach entails the specification of a set of critical values that define appropriate continuation and stopping regions and that guarantee the desired type I and type II error probabilities under repeated significance testing.

Table 3.3 (*Continued*)

- The critical values for early stopping in favour of H_1 will be of the form $b_j^1 = C_1(\alpha, \beta, K, \Delta)j^\Delta$, while critical values for early stopping in favour of H_0 will be of the form $b_j^0 = j\delta^* - C_2(\alpha, \beta, K, \Delta)j^\Delta$, where C_1 and C_2 are positive constants and $b_j^0 \le b_j^1$.
- C_1 and C_2 depend on the required significance level α, the size of the type II error β, the maximum number of looks, K, and an additional parameter Δ that affects the shape of the continuation region. If $\Delta = 0$, the O'Brien–Fleming boundary is obtained. If $\Delta = 0.5$, the Pocock boundary results. More generally, Wang and Tsiatis (1987) explore the family of boundaries to find the value of Δ that minimises the expected sample size for various design specifications.
- The following stategy can be adopted for a one-sided test

$$\text{continue the trial if } S_j \in (b_j^0, b_j^1)$$

- At any analysis, values of $S_j \ge b_j^1$ will be considered supportive of the alternative, while values of $S_j \le b_j^0$ will be considered as supportive of the null, and in either case, the trial will terminate.
- The value of n can be shown to be

$$n = 2\frac{\sigma^2(C_1 + C_2)^2 K^{2(\Delta-1)}}{\delta^2}$$

- The values of C_1 and C_2 that satisfy the required operating characteristics are found using the recursive integration formula described in Armitage *et al.* (1969).

(This account summarises that given in Pampallona and Tsiatis, 1993.)

obtained with the standard. From previous experience, the standard deviation of blood pressure measurements among target patients is of the order of 15 mmHg. The trial is required to have a power of 90% in order to detect the difference of interest when two-sided significance testing is performed at the 5% level. The O'Brien–Fleming boundary, when the number of looks is set at five, is shown in Fig. 3.7. This approach requires a maximum of 102 patients; a fixed sample size design requires 95 patients, but without the possibility of early stopping.

Table 3.4. Values of C_1, C_2 and n for various combinations of β, K and Δ when $\delta/\sigma = 1$ (part of table in Pampallona and Tsiatis, 1994).

K	Δ	$1-\beta = 0.80$ C_1	C_2	n	$1-\beta = 0.80$ C_1	C_2	n
One sided test, $\alpha = 0.05$							
4	0.0	3.3118	1.9987	3.52	3.3722	2.7506	4.69
	0.1	2.9227	1.7954	3.67	2.9760	2.4440	4.85
	0.2	2.6000	1.6225	3.88	2.6454	2.1881	5.08
	0.3	2.3395	1.4748	4.18	2.3766	1.9771	5.44
	0.4	2.1340	1.3479	4.59	2.1635	1.8043	5.97
	0.5	1.9756	1.2383	5.16	1.9981	1.6639	6.71
5	0.0	3.7217	2.2693	2.87	3.7928	3.1052	3.81
	0.1	3.2162	1.9973	3.00	3.2775	2.7012	3.95
	0.2	2.8023	1.7718	3.19	2.8537	2.3698	4.16
	0.3	2.4730	1.5845	3.46	2.5141	2.1021	4.48
	0.4	2.2185	1.4279	3.85	2.2502	1.8883	4.97
	0.5	2.0268	1.2962	4.42	2.0504	1.7189	5.68

It is, of course, possible that use of some suggested procedures for interim analyses will lead to inconsistencies. Falissard and Lellouch (1991), for example, consider a trial planned with four interim analyses and a final one, each analysis occurring after a constant number of patients in each group. A z test for assessing the difference in treatment means is scheduled for each of the five planned analyses, the overall type I error required being 5%. Pocock's method rejects the null hypothesis if for at least one value of i, $i = 1, \ldots, 5$, $|z_i| \geq 2.41$. Now suppose that the results are $|z_i| < 2.41$ for $i = 1, \ldots 4$ and $z_5 = 2.20$. An investigator using no interim analyses will reject the null hypothesis, while one using Pocock's procedure will accept it. Thus, the two investigators will reach different conclusions with exactly the same data. Falissard and Lellouch (1991) propose a new approach which eliminates some of these inconsistencies. This requires, for rejecting the null hypothesis, that a succession of r tests are significant at the current α level. The value of r is chosen so that the global type I error is also near to α.

If interim analyses are to be part of a clinical trial, the investigator planning the trial needs to consider both how many such analyses there should be and how many patients need to be evaluated between successive analyses. These questions are considered in detail by Pocock (1983) and McPherson (1982). These authors also provide tables showing power and expected sample sizes for trials with various numbers of planned interim analyses. For large values of the treatment difference, the expected sample size is considerably reduced by many interim analyses. In most trials, however, such large differences are unlikely, and in these circumstances, Pocock (1983) suggests that there is little statistical advantage in having a large number of repeated significance tests. As a general rule, Pocock recommends a maximum of five interim analyses.

Interim analyses are designed to avoid continuing a trial beyond the point when the accumulated evidence indicates a clear treatment difference. As commented above, this is clearly ethically desirable. But Pocock (1992) suggests that there is a real possibility that interim analyses claiming significant treatment differences will tend to exaggerate the true magnitude of the treatment effect and that often, subsequent analyses (where performed) are likely to show a reduction in both the significance and magnitude of these differences. His explanation of these phenomena is that interim analyses are often timed (either deliberately or unwittingly) to reflect a 'random high' in the treatment comparison. Simon (1994) also makes the point that estimates of treatment effects will be biased in clinical trials which stop early.

Even though group sequential methods can be used to help decide when a trial should be stopped, the subsequent estimation of the treatment effect and its associated p-value still needs careful consideration. It is not difficult to find examples of trials in which some

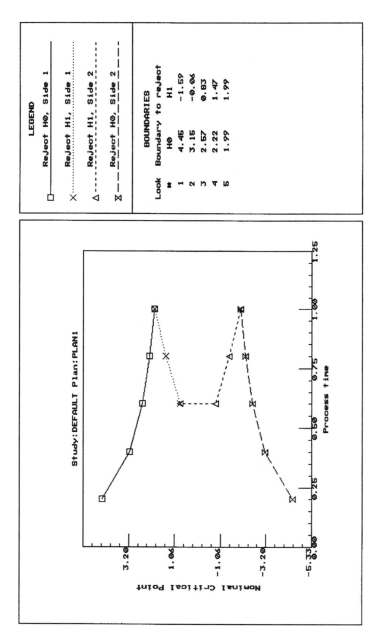

Fig. 3.7.   O'Brien-Fleming boundary obtained from EaSt software for blood pressure example.

type of interim analysis was used to stop the trial early, but where the reported treatment effect estimate and its p-value were not adjusted for the sequential design but instead calculated as if the trial had been of fixed size (see, for example, Moertel *et al.*, 1990). Souhami (1994) suggests that stopping early because an effect is undoubtedly present may result in a serious loss of precision in estimation, and lead to imprecise claims of benefit or detriment. Methods that attempt to overcome such problems are described in Whitehead (1986), Rosner and Tsiatis (1989), Jennison and Turnbull (1989) and Pinheiro and DeMets (1997).

It was the Greenburg Report, finalised in 1967 but not published until 1988, that established the rationale for interim analyses of accumulating data. In addition, however, it emphasised the need for independent data monitoring committees to review interim data and take into consideration the multiple factors that are usually involved before early termination of a clinical trial can be justified. Such factors include baseline comparability, treatment compliance, outcome ascertainment, benefit to risk ratio, and public impact. This type of committee is now regarded as an almost essential component of a properly conducted clinical trial and helps to ensure that interim analyses, by whatever method, do not become overly prescriptive.

3.4.1. Group Sequential Procedures — A Bayesian Perspective

Any discussion of group sequential procedures would be incomplete without acknowledging that some statisticians consider the whole approach almost fatally flawed. Freedman *et al.* (1994), for example, find reason for concern in three areas:

- philosophical awkwardness,
- how to draw inferences if the stopping rule is not followed,
- how to estimate treatment effects at the end of a group sequential trial.

Freedman *et al.* (1994) illustrate their philosophical difficulties with the usual frequentist approaches to interim analyses with the following (hypothetical) situation:

Suppose that a clinician Dr. C comes to statistician Dr. S for some advice. Dr. C has conducted a clinical trial of a new treatment for AIDS. He has treated and assessed 200 patients, and analysis of the results suggests a benefit from the new treatment that is statistically significant ($p = 0.02$). Dr. S, who is also a frequentist, asks how many times Dr. C plans to analyse the results as the trial progresses. We now consider two possible responses.

(1) Dr. C may respond that this is the first and only analysis that has and will be done. He has waited until the data are complete before analysing them. Dr. S is then prepared to endorse the analysis and p-value.

(2) Dr. C may, instead, respond that he intends to include 1000 patients in this trial, and that this is the first of five analyses that are planned. Moreover, the statistician who helped to design the trial had advocated an O'Brien and Fleming boundary. Dr. S then advises Dr. C that the results are not yet statistically significant and that the p-value of 0.02 should not be taken at face value, being one of a series of tests that are planned.

Freedman *et al.* (1994) complain that it seems unreasonable that different inferences should be made by Dr. S depending upon the plan for further analysis. They then suggest an alternative Bayesian approach involving the following steps:

- A prior distribution, representing one's pre-trial belief about the treatment difference is specified. (In fact two priors are recommended, the first to represent a reasonable sceptic, the second to represent a reasonable enthusiast.)
- Data are then gathered during the trial leading to an estimate of the treatment difference with a confidence interval.
- Bayes' theorem is then applied to calculate a posterior distribution that represents one's current belief about the treatment difference.

- Recommendations regarding the continuation of the trial are based upon the posterior distribution. The treatment difference scale is divided into three ranges:

  (1) differences that would lead to a choice of the standard treatment,

  (2) differences that would lead to a choice of the new treatment,

  (3) an intermediate range in which benefits from the new treatment are balanced by increased toxicity, inconvenience or cost.

The posterior probabilitites of the treatment effect lying within each of these three regions may be used to make decisions about the future of the trial. Freedman *et al.* (1994) provide an example of such an approach in a clinical trial investigating the effect of drug combination of 5-flurouracil and levamisole upon the length of survival of patients with colorectal cancer.

Although the properties of the Bayesian approach are attractive in providing an integrated view of all aspects of stopping, it has, so far, failed to make a major impact on monitoring clinical trials. Machin (1994) suggests that this may be partly due to clinicians scepticism over the way that different priors purporting to represent belief, can influence the interpretation of results. He suggests that if the Bayesian approach is to evolve into a more than interesting but unused tool, there is a need for 'case' studies to illustrate what it gives above and beyond current methods. More detailed discussion of Bayesian methods is taken up in Chapter 9.

3.5. SUMMARY

Once a trial begins, a patient's progress needs to monitored closely. Much effort needs to be put into determining whether or not the patient is complying with the intended treatment and trying, wherever, possible to ensure that the patient is observed on all the occasions specified in the trial protocol. The analysis of longitudinal data from a clinical trial which has a substantial proportion of missing values, whilst possible with particular statistical techniques, does present considerably more problems than when the data is complete. The proportion of missing values in a set of data can often legitimately be taken as an indicator of the quality of the study.

The standard way of dealing with non-compliance is intention-to-treat analysis. Only analysis by intention-to-treat can be relied on to provide an unbiased comparison of the treatment *policies* as implemented. All other analyses deviate from the principle of randomised comparison, need to make assumptions that cannot be fully validated and hence carry a risk of introducing bias. Schwartz and Lellouch (1967) characterise trials intended for comparing the efficacy of treatment regimens, 'pragmatic', and for such trials intention-to-treat is the only correct analysis.

But in many cases, interest may be more in comparing the drugs involved in the regimens, what Schwartz and Lellouch label 'explanatory trials'. In this situation, *supplementary* analyses using compliance information recorded for each patient become acceptable. Indeed Efron (1998) suggests that taking into account the variable compliance in a randomised clinical trial may offer advantages such as the derivation of a dose-response curve for the drugs efficacy, even though the original experiment was only intended as a single dose.

The basis of the analyses which are eventually applied to the trial data are the measurements of the outcome variable(s) specified in the trial protocol. Clearly, the quality of the trial can only be as good as the quality of the data collected and issues of the reliability of the chosen outcome measure may need to be addressed.

Continuing a clinical trial beyond the time when there is strong evidence of a substantial treatment difference is ethically undesirable and interim analyses which may allow the trial to be terminated early are usually written into the protocol of the trial. The statistical-based boundaries that result are often quite helpful but should not be viewed as absolute decision rules. In addition, such analyses need to be used with caution since they can lead to over optimistic claims about the effectiveness of treatments in some situations.

CHAPTER 4

Basic Analyses of Clinical Trials, the Generalised Linear Model and the Economic Evaluation of Trials

4.1. INTRODUCTION

Senn (1997) makes the point that in its simplest form a clinical trial consists of a head to head comparison of a single treatment and a control in order to answer a single well defined question. The analysis of such a trial might then consist of applying a single significance test or constructing a single confidence interval for the treatment difference. In practice, of course, matters tend to be a little more complex and most clinical trials generate a large amount of data; for example, apart from the observations of the chosen outcome variable(s) at different points in time, details of side effects, measurements of laboratory safety variables, demographic and clinical covariates will often also be collected. As a consequence, the analyses needed may rapidly increase in complexity. In this chapter we shall restrict attention to methods suitable for trials in which one or more outcome variables are recorded on a single occasion, usually the end of the trial. Later analysis chapters will deal with the more

involved techniques needed to analyse data from trials in which outcome measures are observed on several occasions post-randomisation
and possibly also pre-randomisation.

4.2.   A BRIEF REVIEW OF BASIC STATISTICS

The basic statistical principles required in the analysis and interpretation of data from many clinical trials are well described in Pocock
(1983) and elsewhere; consequently, we shall give only a very brief
review of these methods in this section.

Analysis of a single continuous outcome variable observed once at
the end of a trial usually begins with some simple plots and diagrams,
e.g. histograms, and box plots. Figures 4.1, and 4.2 illustrate each

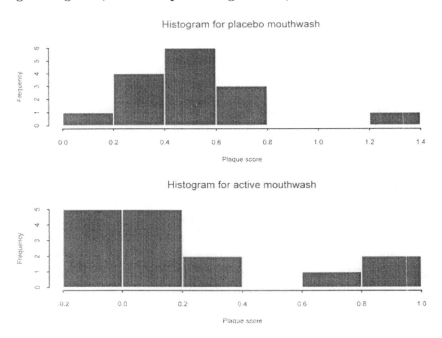

Fig. 4.1. Histograms for placebo and active treatment groups in double-
blind trial of an oral mouthwash.

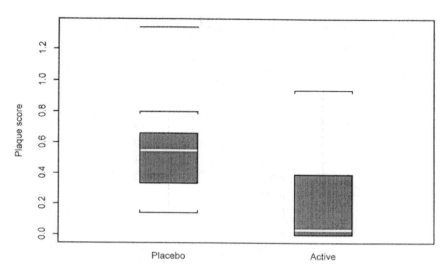

Fig. 4.2. Boxplots for placebo and active treatment groups in double-blind trial of an oral mouthwash.

type of plot for the data shown in Table 4.1; these data arise from a double blind trial in which an oral mouthwash was compared with a placebo mouthwash. Fifteen subjects were randomly allocated to each mouthwash and at the end of 15 weeks an average plaque score was obtained for each subject. This was calculated by allocating a score of 0, 1, 2 or 3 to each tooth and averaging over all teeth present in the mouth. The scores of 0, 1, 2 and 3 for each tooth corresponded, respectively to:

- 0 — no plaque,
- 1 — a film of plaque visible only by disclosing,
- 2 — a moderate accumulation of deposit visible to the naked eye,
- 3 — an abundance of soft matter.

The histogram and boxplot for the placebo group show clear evidence of an outlier, and the corresponding plots for the active group

Table 4.1. Data from Mouthwash Trial.

	Subject	Plaque Score		Subject	Plaque Score
Placebo	1	0.709	*Active*	16	0.000
	2	0.339		17	0.000
	3	0.596		18	0.344
	4	0.333		19	0.059
	5	0.550		20	0.937
	6	0.800		21	0.024
	7	0.596		22	0.033
	8	0.589		23	0.000
	9	0.458		24	0.019
	10	1.339		25	0.687
	11	0.143		26	0.000
	12	0.661		27	0.136
	13	0.275		28	0.000
	14	0.226		29	0.395
	15	0.435		30	0.917

indicate the skewness of the distribution. Despite these contraindications, the data will first be analysed using a two-sample t-test; the results, shown in Table 4.2, suggest that the active mouthwash has been successful in lowering the plaque score.

The indication of non-normality for the mouthwash trial data given by Figs. 4.1 and 4.2, may suggest to some investigators the need to transform the data in some way before applying the t-test; alternatively, a nonparametric test of the treatment difference might be considered appropriate. The question of transformations will be taken up later, but applying the Wilcoxon rank-sum test gives a p-value of 0.001, again clearly demonstrating a non-zero treatment difference (in terms of the two medians). Section 4.5.4 illustrates another approach for dealing with non-normality that uses bootstrap estimation.

In many clinical trials, the outcome variable will be binary. An example is shown in Table 4.3. This arises from a study testing

Table 4.2. Results from Applying Two-sample *t*-test to Mouthwash Data in Table 4.1.

	Placebo	Active
Mean	0.5348	0.2367
SD	0.2907	0.3432
n	15	15

$t = 2.567$, d.f. $= 28$, p-value $= 0.0159$, 95% confidence interval for treatment difference $(0.060, 0.536)$.

Table 4.3. Aspirin and Cardiovascular Disease.

	Myocardial Infarction		
Group	Yes	No	Total
Placebo	189	10,845	11,034
Aspirin	104	10,933	11,037

whether regular intake of aspirin reduces mortality from cardiovascular disease. Every other day, physicians participating in the study took either one aspirin tablet or a placebo. The participants were blind to which type of pill they were taking.

Such data will often be analysed based on a confidence interval for the difference in the population proportions of myocardial infarctions in the aspirin and placebo groups. Details are given in Table 4.4. The derived confidence interval does not contain the value zero and suggests that aspirin diminishes the risk of myocardial infarction.

A further measure of the treatment difference often used for binary outcomes is the *odds ratio*; its calculation for the aspirin data is outlined in Table 4.5. The associated confidence interval does not contain the value one, again indicating the positive effect of aspirin in preventing myocardial infarction. As we shall see later, the odds

Table 4.4. Constructing a Confidence Interval for the Difference in Proportions of Myocardial Infarctions amongst Patients given Aspirin and Placebo.

Of the 11 034 physicians taking placebo, 189 suffered from myocardial infarction over the course of the study, a proportion $p_1 = 189/11034 = 0.0171$.

Of the 11 037 physicians taking aspirin, 104 suffered from myocardial infarction over the course of the study, a proportion $p_2 = 104/11037 = 0.00094$

The sample difference of proportions is $0.0171 - 0.0094 = 0.0077$. This difference has an estimated standard error of

$$\sqrt{\frac{(0.017)(0.9829)}{11034} + \frac{(0.0094)(0.9906)}{11037}} = 0.0015$$

A 95% confidence interval for the true difference is $0.0077 \pm 1.96\,(0.0015)$, i.e., $(0.005, 0.011)$.

Table 4.5. Odds Ratio for Aspirin Study.

For the physicians taking placebo, the estimated odds of myocardial infarction equal $189/10845 = 0.0174$.

For the physicians taking aspirin, the estimated odds of myocardial infarction equal $104/10933 = 0.0095$.

The sample odds ratio $\hat{\theta} = 0.0174/0.0095 = 1.832$. The estimated odds of myocardial infarction for physicians taking placebo equal 1.832 times the estimated odds for physicians taking aspirin. The estimated odds are 83% higher in the placebo group.

The asymptotic standard error of $\log(\hat{\theta})$ is calculated as

$$SE[\log(\hat{\theta})] = \sqrt{\frac{1}{189} + \frac{1}{10933} + \frac{1}{10845} + \frac{1}{104}}$$
$$= 0.123$$

Consequently a 95% confidence interval for $\log \theta$ is $\log(1.832) \pm 1.96\,(0.123)$, i.e., $(0.365, 0.846)$. The corresponding confidence interval for θ is $[\exp(0.365), \exp(0.846)] = (1.44, 2.33)$.

Table 4.6. Pain Scores after Wisdom Tooth Extraction.

Method 1			Method 2		
Patient ID	Age	Pain Score	Patient ID	Age	Pain Score
1	27	36	11	44	20
2	32	45	12	26	35
3	23	56	13	20	47
4	28	34	14	27	30
5	30	30	15	48	29
6	35	40	16	21	45
7	22	57	17	32	31
8	27	38	18	22	49
9	25	45	19	22	25
10	24	49	20	20	39

ratio is a fundamental parameter in particular types of models for binary response variables.

Even in these clinical trials in which comparing two groups with respect to a single outcome variable is of prime interest, we may still wish to take one or more other variables into consideration in the analysis. In particular, if there is a variable known in advance to be strongly related to the chosen outcome measure, taking it into account using *analysis of covariance* can often increase the precision with which the treatment effect can be estimated. To illustrate a simple application of analysis of covariance, the data in Table 4.6 will be used. These arise from a randomised trial of two different methods of wisdom tooth extraction, in which the outcome variable was a measure of pain on discharge derived from a visual analogue scale with anchor points, 0 = no pain and 50 = unbearable pain. The age of each patient was also recorded as it was thought that age would be related to a patient's perception of their pain. A plot of the data is shown in Fig. 4.3.

Details of the analysis of covariance are given in Table 4.7. A simple regression model is assumed in which, conditional on treatment and age, the pain outcome variable is normally distributed with

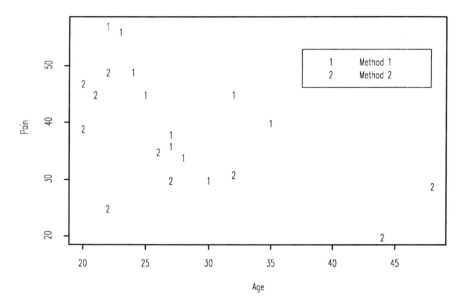

Fig. 4.3. Scatterplot of age of patient vs. pain score after wisdom tooth extraction with patients labelled by treatment group.

constant variance. The results of the analysis indicate that pain is indeed related to age and that the mean pain scores after adjusting for age differ significantly.

(Particularly commonly used covariates in clinical trials are baseline, pre-treatment values of the main response variable; discussion of such covariates is taken up in detail in the next chapter.)

Covariates such as age, etc., may also often be of interest when the outcome variable is binary. But using the linear model given in Table 4.7 for say, the probability of a zero response (P), immediately runs into difficulties. The most obvious is that it could lead to parameter estimates which give fitted probability values outside the range $(0, 1)$. A further problem is that the assumed normal distribution would now clearly not be realistic. Because of these problems,

Table 4.7. Analysis of Covariance of Pain Data in Table 4.6.

The analysis of covariance model assumes that pain on discharge and age are linearly related and that the slope of the regression line is the same for each extraction method. Specifically the model has the form:

$$E(\text{pain}) = \beta_0 + \beta_1 \text{ group} + \beta_2 \text{ age}$$

where group is a dummy variable taking the value 0 for method 1 and the value 1 for method 2. The estimated parameter values and their standard errors are:

variable	parameter	standard error of	estimate/SE
age	−0.74	0.23	3.16
group	−7.33	3.45	2.13

some suitable transformation of the probability is modelled as a linear function of the covariates rather than the probability itself. The most commonly used transformation is the *logistic*, i.e., $\lambda = \ln \frac{P}{1-P}$, leading to *logistic regression*. In addition a more suitable distributional assumption is made.

The linear model used in the analysis of covariance of a normally distributed response and the logistic regression model for binary outcomes are unified along with models for other types of response variables under the *generalised linear model* to which we now turn our attention.

4.3. GENERALISED LINEAR MODELS

The binary response variable is an extreme example of departure from normality for which the linear model described in Table 4.7 is clearly unsuitable. But in the case of more moderate departures from this condition, the model has often been applied to some transformed value assumed to comply with the requirements of approximate conditional normality, linearity and constant variance. Many outcome

measures in common use are, however, resistant to successful transformation. In other cases, the original scale may be a natural one
and effect estimates and inference are more easily understood on this
scale. Measures such as counts of events or symptoms, for example,
typically possess highly skewed distributions where the modal value
is zero or close to it, and do not transform satisfactorily. (Lindsey, 1993, draws a distinction between *frequency* data, obtained by a
classification of sample units typically considered to be independent,
and *count* data obtained as a response from each sample unit and
typically representing a number of events over a period or features
on a surface.) Such measures can, however, often be readily analysed by a model in which the log of the expected count is related to
treatment and covariates with observed counts being assumed Poisson distributed (or Poisson-like — see later) around this expected
value, a model known as *Poisson regression.*

Both logistic regression and Poisson regression are special cases
of a wider class of generalised linear models or GLMs. The models
are described in detail in McCullagh and Nelder (1989) and more
concisely in Table 4.8. The essential features are the link and variance
functions; these are detailed for a variety of GLMs in Table 4.9.
Maximum likelihood estimation of the parameters in such models is
fully described in McCullagh and Nelder (1989) but typically consists
of an iterative weighted least squares solution to the *score equations,*
i.e., the derivatives of the log-likelihood with respect to the regression
parameters. These equations can be written thus:

$$U(\beta) = \sum_{i=1}^{n} \left(\frac{\partial \mu_i}{\partial \beta}\right)' v_i^{-1}\{Y_i - \mu_i(\beta)\} = 0 \qquad (4.1)$$

where v_i^{-1} are weights derived from the variance function $v_i = \mathrm{Var}(Y_i)$. The large sample covariance matrix of the parameter estimates is given by the inverse of the Hessian matrix, $\mathbf{H}(\beta)$, given
by

$$\mathbf{H}(\beta) = \sum_{i=1}^{n} \left(\frac{\partial \mu_i}{\partial \beta}\right)' v_i^{-1} \left(\frac{\partial \mu_i}{\partial \beta}\right) \qquad (4.2)$$

Table 4.8. Components of GLMs.

- The observed data $y_1, \ldots, y_n$ are assumed to be a realisation of random variables $Y_1, \ldots, Y_n$.

- The analysis of covariance model described in Table 4.7 is a simple example of the general linear regression model with p covariates which can be written as:

$$E(Y) = \beta_1 x_1 + \cdots + \beta_p x_p$$

  where $\beta_1, \ldots, \beta_p$ are parameters that have to be estimated from the data.

- For a sample of n observations, the model can be conveniently written as:

$$E(Y) = X\beta$$

  where $Y' = [Y_1, \ldots, Y_n]$, $\beta' = [\beta_1, \ldots, \beta_p]$ and X is the model matrix containing covariate values (usually including a constant to allow estimation of an intercept) for the n observations in the sample.

- Letting $\mu = E(Y)$, the model and its distributional assumptions can be written concisely as:

$$E(Y) = \mu \quad \text{where} \quad \mu = X\beta$$

  and the response variables are normal with constant variance σ^2.

- The model is generalised by first allowing some transformation of the μ_is to be a linear function of the covariates, i.e.,

$$\eta = X\beta$$

  where $\eta_i = g(\mu_i)$ with $g(\cdot)$ being known as the *link function*. Link functions are monotone increasing, and hence invertible; the inverse link $f = g^{-1}$ is an equivalent and often a more convenient function for relating μ to the covariates.

- So for a binary variable, g would be the logit function with $\eta_i = \log(\frac{\mu_i}{1-\mu_i})$ leading to logistic regression. The inverse link is $\mu_i = \frac{e_i^\eta}{1+e_i^\eta}$. This guarantees that μ_i is in the interval $[0, 1]$, which is appropriate since μ_i is an expected proportion or probability in this case.

Table 4.8. (*Continued*)

- The second generalisation of the usual Gaussian regression model is an extended distributional assumption in which the response variables are assumed to have a distribution in the exponential family, having the form:

$$f(y; \theta, \phi) = \exp\{(y\theta - b(\theta))/a(\phi) + c(y, \phi)\}$$

for some specific functions $a(\cdot), b(\cdot)$ and $c(\cdot)$.

- For the normal distribution, for example, $\theta = \mu, \phi = \sigma^2$ and

$$a(\phi) = \phi, \quad b(\theta) = \theta^2/2 \quad c(y, \phi) = -\frac{1}{2}\{y^2/\sigma^2 + \log(2\pi\sigma^2)\}$$

- One aspect of the choice of distribution for a GLM that is fundamental to estimation and inference is the *variance function*, $V(\mu)$, that captures how the variance of the response variable Y depends upon the mean, $\text{Var}(Y) = \phi V(\mu)$ where ϕ is a constant. For the normal distribution, for example, the variance does not depend on the mean and $V(\mu) = 1, \phi = \sigma^2$. For the Poisson distribution the variance is equal to the mean and $V(\mu) = \mu$.

Table 4.9. Parameterisations of Mean and Variance Functions of Various GLMs.

	Normal	Poisson	Binomial	Gamma	Inverse Gaussian
Notation	$N(\mu, \sigma^2)$	$P(\mu)$	$B(m, \pi)/m$	$G(\mu, \nu)$	$IG(\mu, \sigma^2)$
Link function	μ	$\exp(\mu)$	$\ln\left(\dfrac{\mu}{1-\mu}\right)$	$\dfrac{1}{\mu}$	$\dfrac{1}{\mu^2}$
Variance function	1	μ	$\mu(1-\mu)$	μ^2	μ^3

The validity of the covariance matrix in Eq. (4.2) depends on the specification of the variance function being correct. An alternative estimator for the covariance matrix that provides a consistent estimate even when the variance function is specified incorrectly is the so-called 'sandwich estimator', $\mathbf{H}^{-1}(\boldsymbol{\beta})\mathbf{H}_1(\boldsymbol{\beta})\mathbf{H}^{-1}(\boldsymbol{\beta})$ where

$$\mathbf{H}_1(\boldsymbol{\beta}) = \sum_{i=1}^{n} \frac{\partial \mu_i}{\partial \boldsymbol{\beta}} v_i^{-1} \{Y_i - \mu_i(\boldsymbol{\beta})\}\{Y_i - \mu_i(\boldsymbol{\beta})\}' v_i^{-1} \frac{\partial \mu_i}{\partial \boldsymbol{\beta}} \qquad (4.3)$$

Commonly referred to as a 'robust' or 'heteroscedastic consistent' parameter covariance matrix, the use of standard errors derived from this matrix and the related confidence intervals and p-values can provide some protection against inadvertent misspecification of the error component of a model. Such protection is, however, reliant on asymptotic theory. In small samples and when the model is not misspecified, this estimator of the parameter covariance matrix can perform worse than the standard estimator (Breslow, 1990). The robust estimator also plays an important role in some of the techniques to be described in the next chapter.

GLMs can be fitted routinely using widely available software — see the Appendix, and considerably enrich the range of models that might be applied to the data from clinical trials, in particular making it possible to consider appropriate models for outcome measures with specific properties. Binary variables, for example, are most often modelled using logistic regression; this estimates effects, and combines the effects of covariates, on the log-odds scale. Among other properties, the log-odds scale is symmetric, ensuring equivalent inference regardless of the coding of the binary response. But when the binary response that is recorded is in fact a truncated count or an interval censored failure event, with 0 representing absence of some clinical feature or event, and 1 representing the presence or occurrence of at least one such feature or event, symmetry may no be longer appropriate. In such cases, the log-log scale is often more suitable. This scale is not symmetric but the parameter estimates relate naturally to the log-response rate and thus this model has strong links with methods for survival analysis which are discussed in Chapter 8.

When binary and count data are presented in grouped form as y positive responses in a total of m responses, a binomial distribution might be expected, provided that the m observations are uncorrelated. In some circumstances, however, this assumption may be suspect. Examples include where the observations are repeated measures on the same individual (a situation to be considered in detail in Chapters 5 and 7), or correspond to sets of patients with each set drawn from, say, one of a number of clinics. In each case the observations are likely to be correlated. Under such circumstances, the variance of the response data is likely to be larger than that expected from the binomial distribution. There are a number of ways that such extra-binomial variation or *overdispersion* can be accounted for. One is a further generalisation of GLMs in which a scale parameter ϕ is introduced (see Table 4.8), and the resulting model estimated by a procedure suggested by Wedderburn (1974) called maximum quasilikelihood. Wedderburn pointed out that the GLM score equation (4.1) could be solved for any choice of link and variance function even when their integral (the *quasilikelihood*) did not actually correspond to a member of the exponential family nor even to a known parametric distribution. McCullagh (1983) showed that the regression estimates obtained from solving the corresponding *quasi-score functions* were approximately normal, with mean β and variance still given by Eq. (4.2). McCullagh and Nelder (1989) propose a simple moment estimator for the scale parameter ϕ (see bottom of Table 4.8) based on the Pearson residuals. (Other possible approaches to overdispersion are described in Collett, 1991.)

Count data that might usually be modelled by Poisson regression can also show overdispersion since rates can vary amongst individuals. Counts of features, such as metastases or events such as seizures occurring in individuals, for example, often show extra-Poisson variation, and consequently are rarely successfully dealt with using simple Poisson regression. Again, a quasilikelihood approach can be used to take account of the overdispersion. Alternatively, a more general parametric model such as the negative binomial can be used.

To clarify the general comments made above and to illustrate the way in which different choices of model can influence the results, we now describe a detailed application of GLMs to a set of clinical trial data.

4.3.1. Models for Counts: the Treatment of Familial Adenomatous Polyposis (FAP) with a Non-Steroidal Anti-Inflammatory Drug

The example data shown in Table 4.10 come from Giardiello *et al.* (1993) and are also reported in Piantadosi (1997). The data relate to a placebo controlled trial of a non-steroidal anti-inflammatory drug in the treatment of FAP. The trial was halted after a planned interim analysis had suggested compelling evidence in favour of the treatment. Here the longitudinal aspects of the trial will be ignored (they will be considered in a later chapter) and we shall concentrate on analysing the count of the number of colonic polyps at 12 months.

A 'spikeplot' of the count data shown in Fig. 4.4 shows considerable skewness and an extreme value. For this outcome, we will compare the results obtained from an approach using ordinary regression applied to the log-count, a transformation that substantially removes the skew, with results from a variety of GLMs, that all use a log-link but make different assumptions as to how the mean and variance are related.

A t-test (with group variances assumed equal) for the treatment difference in log-count gives the value -3.34; the point estimate of the treatment difference is -1.58 and the associated 95% confidence interval is $(-2.58, -0.58)$. (This is equivalent to the application of a Gaussian regression model with treatment group as the only covariate.) Introducing log-baseline count as a covariate again using the ordinary Gaussian analysis of covariance regression model described in Table 4.7, gives the estimate and confidence interval shown in the first row of Table 4.11. These show the expected increase in precision

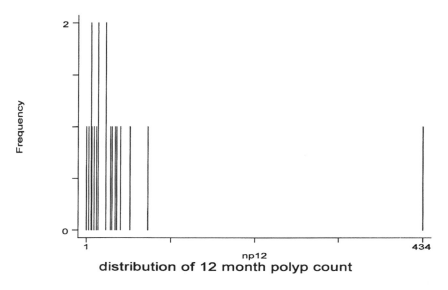

Fig. 4.4.   Spikeplot of count data from a trial of non-steroidal anti-inflammatory drug in the treatment of FAP.

obtainable from baseline covariate adjustment. The point estimates in the other three rows of Table 4.11 are roughly comparable, since they are all estimated on the same log scale. They differ, however, in terms of the variance functions assumed (see Table 4.9) and this will be reflected in the standardised residuals, $(y_i - \hat{\mu}_i)/\sqrt{\text{Var}(\hat{\mu}_i)}$, obtainable after fitting each model. Probability plots of these residuals may help in identifying the most appropriate (and least appropriate) models for these data. Such plots are given in Fig. 4.5. This figure shows the plots corresponding to the four models fitted in Table 4.11 and, in addition, residuals from a Gaussian regression model for the *raw* counts and a standard Poisson regression.

The residuals from the ordinary regression of the raw counts show the failure of this approach to account for the skewness in the data, while those from the standard Poisson regression show a much greater variation than that expected under the assumption that the polyps represented 'independent' events. Uncorrected use of this

Table 4.10. Data from Polyposis CTE Clinical Trial (taken with permission from Piantadosi, 1998).

	Number of Polyps Visit					Size of Polyp Visit							
ID	1	2	3	4	5	1	2	3	4	5	Surg	Age	Treat
1	0	7	6	·	·	·	3.6	3.4	·	·	·	1	17	1
2	0	77	67	71	63	·	3.8	2.8	3.0	2.8	·	1	20	0
3	1	7	4	4	2	4	5.0	2.6	1.2	0.8	1.0	1	16	1
4	0	5	5	16	28	26	3.4	3.6	4.0	2.8	2.1	1	18	0
5	1	23	16	8	17	16	3.0	1.9	1.0	1.0	1.2	1	22	1
6	0	35	31	65	61	40	4.2	3.1	5.6	4.6	4.1	1	13	0
7	0	11	6	1	1	14	2.2	·	0.4	0.2	3.3	1	23	1
8	1	12	20	7	7	16	2.0	2.6	2.2	2.2	3.0	1	34	0
9	1	7	7	11	15	11	4.2	5.0	5.0	3.7	2.5	1	50	0
10	1	318	347	405	448	434	4.8	3.9	5.6	4.4	4.4	1	19	0
11	1	160	142	41	25	26	5.5	4.5	2.0	1.3	3.5	1	17	1
12	0	8	1	2	3	7	1.7	0.4	0.6	0.2	0.8	1	23	1
13	1	20	16	37	28	45	2.5	2.3	2.7	3.2	3.0	1	22	0
14	1	11	20	13	10	32	2.3	2.8	3.7	4.3	2.7	1	30	0
15	1	24	26	55	40	80	2.4	2.2	2.5	2.7	2.7	1	27	0
16	1	34	27	29	33	34	3.0	2.3	2.9	2.5	4.2	1	23	1
17	0	54	45	22	46	38	4.0	4.5	4.2	3.6	2.9	1	22	0
18	1	16	10	·	·	·	1.8	1.0	·	·	·	1	13	1
21	1	30	30	40	50	57	3.2	2.7	3.6	4.4	3.7	0	34	0
22	0	10	6	3	3	7	3.0	3.0	0.6	1.1	1.1	0	23	1
23	0	20	5	1	1	1	4.0	1.1	0.6	0.4	0.4	0	22	1
24	1	12	8	3	4	8	2.8	1.1	0.1	0.4	1.0	0	42	1

Missing values are indicated by a period.

latter model would have led to grossly exaggerated levels of precision and significance for the parameter estimates. The residual plot from the gamma model looks to be the best of the remaining four plots.

More can be learnt about the fit of these four models by considering a further diagnostic, namely the *delta-beta* ($\Delta\beta$) measure of

Table 4.11. Results of Fitting GLMs to Polyposis Data.

Model including baseline	Treatment Effect	z-test	95% CI
Regression of log-count	-1.42	-4.02	$(-2.16, -0.69)$
Overdispersed Poisson	-1.43	-4.69	$(-2.03, -0.83)$
Gamma	-1.25	-5.11	$(-1.74, -0.77)$
Inverse Gaussian	-1.26	-4.54	$(-1.81, -0.72)$

influence proposed by Pregibon (1981) and Williams (1987). This is an example of a *single case deletion diagnostic* that measures the impact of a particular observation on a specific parameter in the model. In general, it is the standardised difference between the parameter estimates with and without a particular observation included. Here our interest will centre on the $\Delta\beta$s associated with the estimated effect of treatment on the log-count of polyps. (The diagnostic is calculated simply by repeated model estimation with each case in turn excluded.)

Index plots of the $\Delta\beta$s for the four models fitted to the polyposis data are shown in Fig. 4.6. The first row of numbers at the top of this plot gives the baseline polyp count used as one of the covariates in the analysis and the second row gives the observed count at the end of 12 months. It is clearly the observation with very low outcome count, namely observation 23 with an outcome of 1, that is most influential in the approach using ordinary regression on the log-counts. Such a finding is not uncommon and cautions against the unquestioning use of the log(1+count) transformation frequently used when zero counts are encountered. For the log-link models, however, this data-point is relatively less influential. Among the log-link models, which points are influential can be understood by a consideration of the mean-variance relationships implied by the choice of error distribution. As can be seen from Table 4.9, the Poisson model assumes the variance to increase in proportion to the mean; for the gamma it increases with the mean squared, while for the inverse-Gaussian it

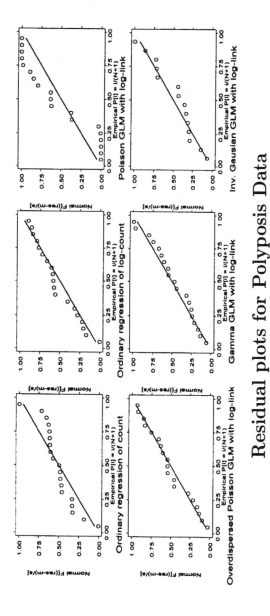

Residual plots for Polyposis Data

Fig. 4.5. Probability plots of residuals from fitting four models to the polyposis data.

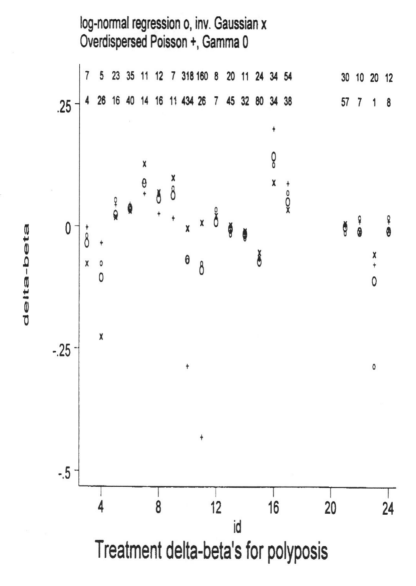

Fig. 4.6. Index plots of delta-beta for the four models fitted to the polyposis data.

increases with the mean cubed. For these data the gamma model, with variance increasing with the mean squared, would seem most appropriate with all the observations having similar and low influence. For the Poisson model, the expected variance of the points with the highest mean (those with the highest baselines) is too small, with these points being attributed greater influence. For the inverse-Gaussian model, the expected variance of those with the lowest means (the lowest baselines) is too small, and correspondingly these points are found to have greater influence.

An alternative way of tackling the problem of non-normal conditional errors using bootstrap is considered in Section 4.5.

4.3.2. Ordinal Response Models: A Clinical Trial in Lymphoma

The data shown in Table 4.12 arise from a clinical trial of cytoxan+prednisone (CP) and BCNU+prednisone (BP) in lymphocytic lymphoma. The outcome variable is the response of the tumour in each patient, measured on a qualitative scale from 'complete response' (best) to 'progression' (worst). It is plausible that this scale represents a unidimensional ordinal scale. A variety of models will now be considered for these data.

Table 4.12. A Clinical Trial in Lymphoma.

	BP	CP	Total
Complete response	26	31	57
Partial response	51	59	110
No change	21	11	32
Progression	40	34	74
Total	138	135	273

4.3.2.1. Models with parallel linear predictors

Two natural extensions of the binary logistic regression model that might be considered for these data are the *proportional-odds model* and the *continuation-ratio model*.

The proportional-odds model can be considered as an extension of the binary logistic model in which, instead of a single threshold partitioning scores on a continuous dimension into two categories, multiple thresholds result in multiple partitions. The log-odds of the probability of falling in any category to the right $(1 - \sum_{j<k} p_{ij})$ and left $(\sum_{j<k} p_{ij})$ of the binary partition, formed by considering each threshold k in turn, is assumed to conform to a model with parallel linear predictors, such that for individual i:

$$\log\left[\sum_{j<k} p_{ij} \Big/ \left(1 - \sum_{j<k} p_{ij}\right)\right] = \alpha_k + \beta' x_i \qquad (4.4)$$

This construction of model fits naturally in circumstances in which pooling of adjacent categories could be plausibly considered. This model is one of many that are based on categories defined by the potentially arbitrary partitioning of a cumulative distribution function. Conceptually, very similar models using the complementary-log-log and probit links are possible.

The continuation ratio model is an alternative model that extends the ordinary logistic model by considering the categories as occurring sequentially, with each advancement to the next category conforming to binary logistic models with parallel linear predictors, but where advancement to the next category is conditional upon having advanced through all previous categories. For this model:

$$\log\left[p_{ik} \Big/ \left(1 - \sum_{j<k} p_{ij}\right)\right] = \alpha_k + \beta' x_i \qquad (4.5)$$

Again, complementary log-log or probit link functions could be used instead of logistic.

4.3.2.2. Non-parallel models

In the preceeding models, only the intercept α varied with the category; the regression coefficients were assumed common. Allowing the regression coefficient to vary with k allows for non-parallel regressions, with effects that apply at some levels but not others. In many applications, the question as to whether parallel linear predictors can be assumed may be an open one. For example, the biochemical action of some drug treatment might be thought likely to interrupt disease progression at one stage transition (threshold) rather than another. The ability to test for heterogeneity in regression coefficients across thresholds may therefore be important. Models with such flexibility are sometimes referred to as partial-proportional models (Peterson and Harrell, 1990).

4.3.2.3. Model estimation

The models described above can be estimated by direct maximum-likelihood using purpose written programs. However, both parallel and non-parallel models can be estimated by forming multiple records for each subject, each record representing the response on each of the notional component binary response models described above. In the case of the proportional odds models and similar models based on the other possible link/cumulative distribution functions, the records from the same individual cannot be considered as independent (Snell, 1964; Clayton, 1974)) but instead form a single multivariate set. There are a number of more and less efficient ways in which this correlation can be accounted for, some of which are considered later. The advantage of this overall approach is that tests of the significance of regression terms involving the interaction between dummy variables for record and predictor variables can be used to test for non-parallel linear predictors.

Figure 4.7 shows the cumulative distribution functions over the ordered response categories for the two treatments for lymphocytic lymphoma. This simple plot suggests there to be rather little difference in the two treatment groups. Fitting an ordinal logistic regression model to these data using maximum likelihood, gave an estimated log-odds ratio of 0.322 in favour of the CP treatment but

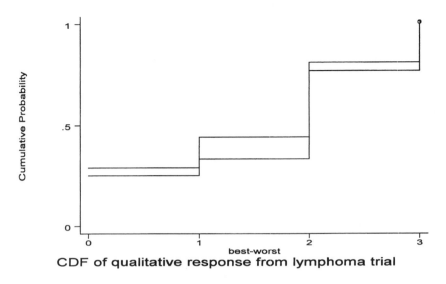

Fig. 4.7. Cumulative distribution functions over the ordered response categories for the two treatments of lymphotic lymphoma.

with a 95% confidence interval from -0.112 to 0.756. The estimate obtained from fitting the same model but specified as a set of three binary logistic regressions (with responses complete versus the rest, complete or partial versus the rest, and the rest versus progression) with different intercepts but common slope, and under the assumption of independence, gave an estimate of 0.314. Of course, the standard errors from such a model will be incorrect, since the three responses will be correlated.

One approach for dealing with this correlation turns out to be remarkably straightforward and will be one that we turn to repeatedly throughout this book. We have already introduced the heteroscedastic consistent/sandwich/robust variance estimator earlier in this chapter. This gave consistent estimates of standard errors even when the chosen model error was inappropriate. The central part of the sandwich defined in Eq. (4.3) assumes independent observations. In our correlated multivariate response context, this can be achieved simply by summing the score contributions within each cluster to form 'super-observations' that are independent. The standard formula can then be applied (Binder, 1983; Rogers, 1993).

Using this robust covariance matrix approach for testing correlated multivariate responses allowed a test for non-parallel linear predictors (non-proportionality in this case), corresponding to whether treatment effects were uniform across all levels of disease severity. The Wald chi-square of 0.10 (p = 0.9) obtained for this 2-degree-of-freedom interaction between treatment and the three severity thresholds, provided no evidence for non-parallel effects. There was little evidence for the treatment effect varying with severity.

A further example of the application of a generalized linear model will be given in Chapter 5.

4.4. MULTIPLE ENDPOINTS

While a small minority of large simple trials may focus on a single outcome measure, for example, mortality, in most circumstances this would be an oversimplification of the diversity of patient response. In many disease conditions, response to treatment can have many different aspects; consequently, clinical trials frequently lack a single definitive outcome measure that completely describes treatment efficacy. When a treatment is thought to affect a disease in a multitude of ways, several outcome variables may be necessary to fully describe its effect on patients. Berkey *et al.* (1996) give an example involving the efficacy of second-line drugs in rheumatoid arthritis (i.e., drugs used after the initial standard therapies are unsuccessful). Efficacy is evaluated on a variety of measures, often including tender joint count, erythrocyte sedimentation rate and grip strength. In general, the multiple outcomes might include clinical events, symptoms, physiological measurements, blood tests, side effects and quality of life.

Pocock (1996) suggests that one possible approach would be the pre-specification of priorities amongst the outcome measures. This would have the result of providing a clear framework for emphasis (and de-emphasis) of results in eventual publication. Such prioritisation is at its simplest when a single outcome measure is selected in advance. As Pocock points out, however, when results actually arrive, it can be difficult to adhere to such principles.

Comparing treatment groups on each of the outcome measures at some chosen significance level α will, as we have seen earlier in this chapter, inflate the type I error. In the unlikely event that the measures are independent, the probability of declaring that at least one is significant when there are in fact no treatment differences is:

$$P = 1 - (1 - \alpha)^m$$

where m is the number of outcome measures. For $\alpha = 0.05$ this leads to:

m	P
1	0.05
2	0.0975
3	0.14625
4	0.18549
5	0.22622
10	0.40126
20	0.64151
50	0.92306

Various procedures have been proposed for keeping the probability that we reject one or more of the true null hypotheses in a set of comparisons (the *familywise error*, FWE) below or equal to a specified level α. The most familar of these is the *Bonferroni procedure* which controls the FWE rate by conducting each test on an outcome measure at level α/m. This is simple to apply but suffers from considerable drawbacks. The first is that it is excessively conservative, particularly if m is large. Consequently, the rather unsatisfactory situation can arise where many tests are significant at level α but none at level α/m. In addition, the Bonferroni correction ignores the degree to which the chosen outcome measures may be correlated, which again leads to conservatism when such correlations are substantial (see Blair *et al.*, 1996). There are alternative approaches which, partially at least, overcome the first problem — see, for example, Holm (1979) and Hochberg (1988). Unfortunately, these alternatives do nothing to address the second problem of correlations between measures. More recently, Blair *et al.* (1996) have described permutational methods which appear to overcome the conservatism problem even in situations with many outcomes which have large correlations.

Even if some appropriate adjustment of p-values could be found there remains the risk of data dredging and distortive reporting by a post hoc emphasis on the most statistically impressive findings.

An alternative to testing each outcome measure separately at a significance level calculated to control the FWE rate, is to use a procedure which *simultaneously* tests for treatment differences on all variables. Such tests take into consideration the empirical correlation structure of the outcome measures, thus overcoming one of the criticisms of methods such as the Bonferroni correction. The most commonly used of these global tests is Hotelling's T^2, which is the multivariate analogue of the two-sample t-test. To test the equality of two mean vectors against the alternative that they differ in some respect, the T^2 statistic is:

$$T^2 = \frac{n_1 n_2}{n} (\bar{\mathbf{x}}_1 - \bar{\mathbf{x}}_2)' \mathbf{S}^{-1} (\bar{\mathbf{x}}_1 - \bar{\mathbf{x}}_2) \tag{4.6}$$

where n_1 and n_2 are the number of observations in the two groups and $n = n_1 + n_2$; $\bar{x}_1$ and $\bar{x}_2$ are the sample mean vectors in each group and $\mathbf{S}$ is the estimate of the assumed common covariance matrix given by:

$$\mathbf{S} = \frac{(n_1 - 1)\mathbf{S}_1 + (n_2 - 1)\mathbf{S}_2}{n_1 + n_2 - 2} \tag{4.7}$$

where $\mathbf{S}_1$ and $\mathbf{S}_2$ are the sample covariance matrices in each group.

Under the equality hypothesis and assuming that the outcome measures have a multivariate normal distribution with the same co-variance matrix in each of the two treatment groups, then:

$$F = (n - m - 1)T^2/(n - 2)m \tag{4.8}$$

has an F distribution with m and $n - m - 1$ degrees of freedom.

As an example of the use of Hotelling's test, it will be applied to the size and log-count outcomes at 12 months in the polyposis data given in Table 4.10. The results are detailed in Table 4.13. The test indicates a significant treatment difference on the bivariate mean of the two variables.

Table 4.13. Hotelling's Test for Log-count and Size Variables at 12 Months in Polyposis Data.

- The variance-covariance matrices of the two treatment groups are;

$$\mathbf{S}_1 = \begin{pmatrix} 1.001 & 0.4903 \\ 0.4903 & 0.5321 \end{pmatrix}$$

$$\mathbf{S}_2 = \begin{pmatrix} 1.1298 & 1.1956 \\ 1.1956 & 1.9975 \end{pmatrix}$$

- The combined estimate of the assumed common covariance matrix is

$$\mathbf{S} = \begin{pmatrix} 1.0162 & 0.8222 \\ 0.8222 & 1.2217 \end{pmatrix}$$

- The sample mean vectors are

$$\bar{\mathbf{x}}_1' = [3.7526, 3.1100]$$
$$\bar{\mathbf{x}}_2' = [2.1726, 1.1833]$$

- These lead to $T^2 = 11.1612$ and $F = 5.2523$. The associated p-value is 0.018.

Although Hotelling's T^2 test accounts for the correlations between the outcome measures, it is not without its own problems. First simultaneous testing of all the outcome variables may not answer a practically relevant problem; it is only really useful when the different variables measure different aspects of the same underlying concept. Second the 'directionless' alternative hypothesis associated with the test may mean that it lacks power. Some alternatives which are more powerful if treatment improves all outcomes are described in Follman (1995).

4.5. ECONOMIC EVALUATION OF TRIALS

Of increasing importance to health service providers are questions that go beyond determining whether new treatments are more effective than the current standard treatment. Among these are questions relating to treatment costs. For example, at its simplest, where a new treatment is quite obviously cheaper than the current standard, then a trial that shows that a new treatment is equivalent in effectiveness to the standard may be sufficient reason to argue for the adoption of the new treatment over the old.

The appeal of economic evaluations of trials is at least two-fold. First, policy makers and accountants immediately find the results of research more interesting and relevant, and thus may be persuaded by them. Secondly, the approach seems to take a disparate set of input and outcome measures and sum them up on a single 'objective' scale, one measured in monetary units. Considerable caution is required on both counts to ensure that real clinical and patient benefits are not overlooked and that the unit costs used as weights in this economic weighted sum are indeed appropriate.

4.5.1. Measuring Costs

In practice routine audit systems rarely give adequate data for a proper evaluation of costs. Thus in practice trials may need to include extended measurement protocols that can provide full treatment costs at the individual patient level. A variety of issues need to be borne in mind when considering these measures:

(1) Defining a cost is surprisingly complex. Are costs borne by patients rather than treatment providers to be included? Time off work might not be, but what about the costs of travel to receive treatment, or costs that are passed on directly from treatment provider to patient?

(2) Some costs are transfer costs and should not be included. Different treatments may involve a transfer in the billing of the same cost from one department to another, with no net change in cost.

(3) Costs should not be included for services that would not have been used elsewhere. For example, consider a new treatment that makes use of some currently rarely used but nonetheless necessary piece of equipment. Provided the use made of this equipment by the new treatment does not conflict with its current use, then much less than the full cost of this equipment should be attributed to the new treatment. The calculation of the appropriate amount, the so-called *marginal opportunity cost*, is often far from straightforward.

(4) Costs should not be counted twice. Thus drug costs charged to patients should not be included in both hospital costs and patient costs.

(5) In the same way that clinical outcomes are monitored and compared for a specified period of time, so too it is the case for costs. Longer term treatment benefits might include lower use, or sometimes greater use, of quite a range of health service facilities for complaints not obviously directly related to that treated. For example, patients with successfully treated heart conditions may experience longer term psychiatric problems that are costly to treat. Are these costs to be included? A further complication is that in most branches of economics it is usual to apply a discount rate to future costs, a reflection of the fact that where costs are deferred interest can be earned on the corresponding funds. What, if any, discount rate should be applied?

As a consequence of issues such as these, costs are easier to define within a small closed economic unit than within a community as a whole and can be substantially different. The cost of a treatment as viewed from the perspective of a single private health care provider can be very different from that viewed from the perspective of a national health service.

The uncertainties as to the inclusion criteria and amounts to assign makes this area of measurement one that should be subject to the same rigours as the rest of the trial protocol. This should include the need to define the range of eligible costs prior to randomisation; the need for blindness in the collection of the economic data; and, particularly where the determination of unit costs are part of the analysis stage (i.e., are not known and agreed prior to the study), the importance of blindness and probably also 'independence' at the data-analysis stage.

4.5.2. Analysis of Cost Data

When it comes to analysis, further considerations need to be borne in mind that relate to how the costs come about.

(1) The first relates to the characteristics of the treatment. In many cases, although treatments are routine, and thus might be considered to have a roughly standard fixed cost, they are routine only for a proportion of patients. For the remainder, a variety of complications and side effects result in the need for repeated, different or additional treatment. As a consequence, the distribution of costs by patient is typically highly skewed, often with a small number of patients accounting for a disproportionate amount of the costs.

(2) Economic costs are a measure where the scale of measurement is fixed and known. As a consequence, analyses that attempt to deal with the non-normality of the cost outcome by transformation are not appropriate. This is because the estimated difference in log-costs (or any other nonlinear transformation) of two treatments is

not the same as the log of the estimated cost difference. The analysis of transformed costs simply does not answer the question of interest. Instead, an approach that analyses the untransformed cost using some appropriate GLM should be used, for example, using a model with gamma or inverse-gaussian distributed errors and log-link function. In such a model, the use of the log-link function means that treatment and other effects are estimated in terms of a multiplicative effect, implying an ability to report findings in terms of a percentage reduction or increase in mean costs. Although slightly less familiar to accountants than reporting an absolute cost difference (which can anyway still be derived), the structure of the model recognizes that costs cannot fall below zero. An alternative approach is to persist in the use of OLS linear model methods that give consistent estimates regardless of the distribution of costs, but to recognize their non-normality by the use of a method such as *bootstrap resampling* to estimate the standard errors. A third approach that may be more helpful when the cost distribution shows signs of bimodality, is to focus attention more directly on the factors, including treatment, that distinguish the high cost from the standard cost individuals, using logistic regression on a binary split of the cost data.

(3) Almost always patient costs are derived by the application of unit costs to data on the number of units used by each patient. The units might include days and nights on an in-patient ward, number of outpatient assessments, units of blood products infused and so on. At least two potentially important consequences follow. Firstly, if there is variation in the costs of the same units between patients it is unlikely that this variation occurs at the patient level, but more often at the level of the medical centre, supplier or some such. Thus, from the point of view of costs, patients may fall within a much more complex sampling design, perhaps with nesting within centre, or within a crossed design of suppliers of different products or services. A failure to recognize such clustering may give a misleading impression as to the

precision in the estimates of costs and cost differences. Secondly, and perhaps more importantly, there is typically considerable uncertainty in the costs of many of the units measured, and since the same unit costs are commonly applied across many or even all of the patients, a different choice of unit cost can substantially alter the overall results of a study. A common response to this problem is to narrow the focus of the analysis merely to those costs that can be well measured. Sometimes such costs represent a trivial proportion of the total costs and to narrow the focus in this way then makes very little sense. An alternative response is to consider a range of values for each unit cost, presenting the results in the form of a sensitivity analysis. This typically provides results of little value, since it is frequently the case that few differences prove to be robust under the whole of the plausible unit cost space. One sensible way to approach this issue would be to formulate sensible distributions for unit costs and then to use these within a simulation-based estimation method (see Chapter 9).

4.5.3. Cost-Benefit Analysis

The previous section makes clear that in the presence of uncertainty, the analysis of cost data from a trial may be far from straightforward. In practice, the economic evaluation of benefits are still more complicated and uncertain than those of costs. Benefits may accrue not only to patients but to patient carers, their partners and families, and to the wider society. Deciding where to draw the line, the placing of monetary values on benefits that may be of such very disparate kinds, and the social equity issues in deciding whose valuations they should be, has persuaded most not to attempt such a project.

4.5.4. An Example: Cognitive Behavioral Therapy

The RCT of cognitive-behavioral therapy for psychosis by Kuipers *et al.*, (1998) is a good example of recent attempts to incorporate an economic perspective into trial evaluation. A subset of the raw data is presented in Table 4.14. In view of the likely novelty of such measures to statisticians, we describe this study in some detail. As mentioned above as a currently common occurrence, the economic evaluation of this trial was not part of the original protocol. Costs during the primary nine-month treatment phase of the study were obtained by applying estimated unit costs to in-patient hospital service utilisation records. This necessarily represented a restricted range of items within the wider cost space that might have been examined, essentially focussing on the direct service costs of the CBT treatment itself over standard treatment. The 9–18 month follow-up phase was more systematically evaluated using a Client Service Receipt Inventory (CSRI; Beecham and Knapp, 1992). This considered a wider range of costs, including some accomodation costs, but did not include informal care-giver support nor potentially illness-related unemployment. Again, cost figures were commonly derived by the application of unit costs, often based on adjustment of national estimates of long-run marginal costs (Netten and Dennett, 1996) rather than actual costs (the latter may have been neither known nor necessarily appropriate).

In common with most community-based trials of severe psychiatric disorder, loss to follow-up represented a considerable problem, made worse by additional non-response to the CSRI, the economic evaluation instrument. The figures of Table 4.15 relate to the 31 out of 60 subjects for whom full cost data could be calculated. Figure 4.8 presents box-plots of the total cost for each treatment group, showing the distributions to have the expected heavier upper tails. Various methods for calculating the cost differential and its confidence interval are shown below. Among these is bootstrap estimation (Efron, 1979) in which the precision of estimators is examined by using their empirical distribution when repeated on many resamplings from the sample actually observed. The new samples are of the same size, but the sampling is done with replacement, and consequently the sample members change from sample to sample. Confidence intervals for

Table 4.14. Estimated Patient Costs from the CBT Trial.
(Kuipers *et al.* 1998 and pers. comm.)

	Group	Estimated Costs Accomod'n	Followup	Treatment	Total
1.	cbt	4953	630	5583	11166
2.	cbt	.	.	.	.
3.	cbt	5589	12372	18261	36522
4.	cbt	6084	2177	8261	16522
5.	cbt	3120	2387	5507	11014
6.	cbt	.	.	.	.
7.	cbt	.	.	.	.
8.	cbt	4680	1044	5724	11448
9.	cbt	.	.	.	.
10.	cbt	.	.	.	.
11.	cbt	5499	21599	27098	54196
12.	cbt	6084	1517	7601	15202
13.	cbt	6162	11460	17622	35244
14.	cbt	7917	352	8269	16538
15.	cbt	.	.	.	.
16.	cbt	8814	270	9084	18168
17.	cbt	.	.	.	.
18.	cbt	6162	438	6600	13200
19.	cbt	7917	1067	8984	17968
20.	cbt	7137	15329	22466	44932
21.	cbt	.	.	.	.
22.	cbt	3120	3811	6931	13862
23.	cbt	4953	109	5062	10124
24.	cbt	7683	1670	9353	18706
25.	cbt	.	.	.	.
26.	cbt	.	3212	.	.
27.	cbt	.	.	.	.
28.	cbt	8814	208	9022	18044
29.	cbt	.	.	.	.
30.	control	.	.	.	.

Table 4.14 (*Continued*)

	Group	Accomod'n	Followup	Treatment	Total
		Estimated Costs			
31.	control	·	·	·	·
32.	control	6162	6645	12807	25614
33.	control	6084	852	6936	13872
34.	control	·	·	·	·
35.	control	·	·	·	·
36.	control	6786	6015	12801	25602
37.	control	11349	4047	15396	30792
38.	control	·	·	·	·
39.	control	5889	2016	7905	15810
40.	control	3120	1742	4862	9724
41.	control	6786	4734	11520	23040
42.	control	4953	1026	5979	11958
43.	control	·	·	·	·
44.	control	5889	12323	18212	36424
45.	control	·	·	·	·
46.	control	·	·	·	·
47.	control	6786	1600	8386	16772
48.	control	·	·	·	·
49.	control	·	·	·	·
50.	control	6162	738	6900	13800
51.	control	7917	2334	10251	20502
52.	control	7059	25383	32442	64884
53.	control	·	·	·	·
54.	control	·	·	·	·
55.	control	6084	21364	27448	54896
56.	control	·	·	·	·
57.	control	·	·	·	·
58.	control	·	·	·	·
59.	control	7137	440	7577	15154
60.	control	·	·	·	·

Table 4.15 Economic Evaluation Of Cognitive Therapy Trial.

	Cost Difference UK-pounds (CBT-control)	95% CI CI
Simple *t*-test (equal variances)	−3912	(−14407, 6583)
Simple *t*-test (unequal variances)	−3912	(−14588, 6765)
Robust GLM (overdispersed gamma)	−3912	(−13782, 5959)
Bootstrap linear regression	−3912	
(1000 samples)		
normal approximation method		(−13917, 6094)
empirical percentile method		(−14002, 5307)
bias-corrected percentile		(−14710, 4962)

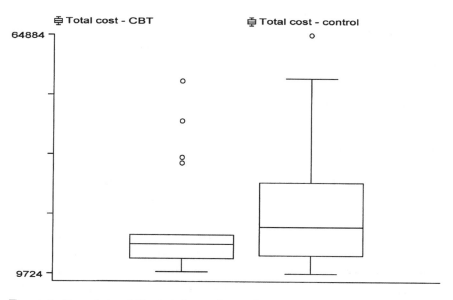

Fig. 4.8. Box-plots of the total cost for each treatment group in the clinical trial of cognitive-behavioural therapy for psychosis.

a parameter estimate can be based on a normal approximation using an estimate of the standard deviation of the empirical distribution, or can be based on the quantiles of the empirical distribution (requiring more samples but not assuming normality). These can also be adjusted to yield so-called bias corrected intervals (Efron and Tibshirani, 1986). Both the GLM and bootstrap percentile methods generate asymmetric intervals reflecting the skew in the cost distributions.

As in many studies some unit costs were easier to measure than others and some represented a substantial proportion of the total cost. In this study, the number of days of inpatient care was relatively easily obtained, sometimes even when patients were non-responders at follow-up. The simple correlation between this variable and total cost was 0.93. Thus this variable by itself might be considered as a useful surrogate for overall cost, with the advantage that it was available for 53 patients rather than just the 32 with total cost data. Analysis of this variable on the larger sample supported the lack of treatment difference in costs, the bootstrap percentile interval for the difference in in-patients days being -32.0 to 7.10. An alternative use for this variable would be to use it to reweight the sample with complete cost data in an attempt to correct for selective loss. This issue is taken up in later chapters.

4.6. SUMMARY

The primary data for analysis in many clinical trials will consist of the observations of one or more outcome variables taken at the end of the trial. In many cases the analysis might consist of the construction of a simple confidence interval appropriate for the type of variable at hand. When covariates other than treatment group are of interest, then it will usually be necessary to consider some form of model for the data. Many investigators often use Gaussian-based regression for all but binary variables, where simple logistic regression is usually applied. But it will frequently be advantageous to consider more carefully the nature of the outcome variable and try to find a more suitable GLM.

One important element in this choice of model is the scale upon which it is desired to estimate effects. For economic data, the scale is clear and one for which a transformation of the response variable would not be helpful. Appropriate choice of GLM or the use of methods such as bootstrap that are based on the empirical distribution were shown to be more suitable. Unlike most clinical measures, the construction of economic measures draws on a considerable amount of information external to the trial. Trial protocols should where possible bring the construction of these measures within their scope. The common practice of using unit costs may also generate complex patterns of correlated measurement error not easily dealt with at the analysis stage.

When multiple endpoints are available a variety of methods might be applied. If the number of outcomes is small, say less than five, then adjusting significance levels using the Bonferroni correction or some less conservative adjustment may suffice. Alternatively, simultaneous inference using Hotelling's test may be required. With a large number of outcome measures the problems become more difficult. In many cases having many outcome measures may be indicative of a poorly thought out study. Pocock (1996) points out the merit in drawing up pre-defined strategies for statistical analysis and reporting of trials with appropriate pre-declaration of priorities, since there is a clear need to safeguard against manipulative *post hoc* emphases and distortions in conclusions. On the other hand, a protocol that is too prescriptive may lead to inflexibility and a supression of both clinical and statistical 'insight'.

CHAPTER 5

Simple Approaches to the Analysis of Longitudinal Data from Clinical Trials

5.1. INTRODUCTION

Medical treatments rarely result in a one time final result for a patient; generally, they require clinicians to follow the evolution of a patient's health over a period of time. Consequently, in the majority of clinical trials the primary outcome variables are observed on several occasions post randomisation and often also prior to randomisation. Such *longitudinal data* can be analysed in a variety of ways. In the last decade, many powerful new methods have been developed which allow a variety of potentially useful models to be applied, many of which can be employed when the data are unbalanced for whatever reasons. (As we shall see in the next two chapters, however, fitting such models to unbalanced data requires considerable care if misleading inferences are to be avoided.) Some of the newly developed techniques are also able to deal with non-normal outcome variables, e.g., binary variables indicating the presence or absence of some characteristic. This methodology will be considered in detail in Chapters 6 and 7.

In this chapter, however, we concentrate on an account of a number of relatively simple approaches to the analysis of longitudinal data. For many studies these methods may provide a perfectly adequate analysis, for whilst simple, they are not necessarily simplistic and are often extremely useful when applied sensibly. Even when they fail to provide the complete answer to the analysis of a set of longitudinal data, they may frequently prove to be useful adjuncts to the more complex modelling procedures to be described later. As with most data analysis situations, graphical displays of the data are an essential preliminary step and this is where we begin.

5.2. GRAPHICAL METHODS FOR DISPLAYING LONGITUDINAL DATA

Graphical displays of data are often useful for exposing patterns in the data, particularly when these are unexpected; this might be of great help in suggesting which class of models might be most sensibly applied in the later more formal analysis. According to Diggle *et al.* (1994), there is no single prescription for making effective graphical displays of longitudinal data, although they do offer the following simple guidelines:

- show as much of the relevant raw data as possible rather than only data summaries;
- highlight aggregate patterns of potential scientific interest;
- identify both cross-sectional and longitudinal patterns;
- make easy the identification of unusual individuals or unusual observations.

A number of graphical displays which can be useful in the preliminary assessment of longitudinal data from clinical trials will now be illustrated using the data shown in Table 5.1. These data arise from a double-blind, placebo controlled trial involving 61 women with major depression, that had begun within 3 months of childbirth and

Table 5.1. Data from Trial of Oestrogen Patch for Treating Post-natal Depression.

Group	BL1	BL2	V1	V2	V3	V4	V5	V6
0	18.00	18.00	17.00	18.00	15.00	17.00	14.00	15.00
0	25.11	27.00	26.00	23.00	18.00	17.00	12.00	10.00
0	19.00	16.00	17.00	14.00	−9.00	−9.00	−9.00	−9.00
0	24.00	17.00	14.00	23.00	17.00	13.00	12.00	12.00
0	19.08	15.00	12.00	10.00	8.00	4.00	5.00	5.00
0	22.00	20.00	19.00	11.54	9.00	8.00	6.82	5.05
0	28.00	16.00	13.00	13.00	9.00	7.00	8.00	7.00
0	24.00	28.00	26.00	27.00	−9.00	−9.00	−9.00	−9.00
0	27.00	28.00	26.00	24.00	19.00	13.94	11.00	9.00
0	18.00	25.00	9.00	12.00	15.00	12.00	13.00	20.00
0	23.00	24.00	14.00	−9.00	−9.00	−9.00	−9.00	−9.00
0	21.00	16.00	19.00	13.00	14.00	23.00	15.00	11.00
0	23.00	26.00	13.00	22.00	−9.00	−9.00	−9.00	−9.00
0	21.00	21.00	7.00	13.00	−9.00	−9.00	−9.00	−9.00
0	22.00	21.00	18.00	−9.00	−9.00	−9.00	−9.00	−9.00
0	23.00	22.00	18.00	−9.00	−9.00	−9.00	−9.00	−9.00
0	26.00	26.00	19.00	13.00	22.00	12.00	18.00	13.00
0	20.00	19.00	19.00	7.00	8.00	2.00	5.00	6.00
0	20.00	22.00	20.00	15.00	20.00	17.00	15.00	13.73
0	15.00	16.00	7.00	8.00	12.00	10.00	10.00	12.00
0	22.00	21.00	19.00	18.00	16.00	13.00	16.00	15.00
0	24.00	20.00	16.00	21.00	17.00	21.00	16.00	18.00
0	−9.00	17.00	15.00	−9.00	−9.00	−9.00	−9.00	−9.00
0	24.00	22.00	20.00	21.00	17.00	14.00	14.00	10.00
0	24.00	19.00	16.00	19.00	−9.00	−9.00	−9.00	−9.00
0	22.00	21.00	7.00	4.00	4.19	4.73	3.03	3.45
0	16.00	18.00	19.00	−9.00	−9.00	−9.00	−9.00	−9.00
1	21.00	21.00	13.00	12.00	9.00	9.00	13.00	6.00
1	27.00	27.00	8.00	17.00	15.00	7.00	5.00	7.00
1	24.00	15.00	8.00	12.27	10.00	10.00	6.00	5.96
1	28.00	24.00	14.00	14.00	13.00	12.00	18.00	15.00

Table 5.1 (*Continued*)

Group	BL1	BL2	V1	V2	V3	V4	V5	V6
1	19.00	15.00	15.00	16.00	11.00	14.00	12.00	8.00
1	17.00	17.00	9.00	5.00	3.00	6.00	0.00	2.00
1	21.00	20.00	7.00	7.00	7.00	12.00	9.00	6.00
1	18.00	18.00	8.00	1.00	1.00	2.00	0.00	1.00
1	24.00	28.00	11.00	7.00	3.00	2.00	2.00	2.00
1	21.00	21.00	7.00	8.00	6.00	6.50	4.64	4.97
1	19.00	18.00	8.00	6.00	4.00	11.00	7.00	6.00
1	28.00	27.46	22.00	27.00	24.00	22.00	24.00	23.00
1	23.00	19.00	14.00	12.00	15.00	12.00	9.00	6.00
1	21.00	20.00	13.00	10.00	7.00	9.00	11.00	11.00
1	18.00	16.00	17.00	26.00	−9.00	−9.00	−9.00	−9.00
1	22.61	21.00	19.00	9.00	9.00	12.00	5.00	7.00
1	24.24	23.00	11.00	7.00	5.00	8.00	2.00	3.00
1	23.00	23.00	16.00	13.00	−9.00	−9.00	−9.00	−9.00
1	24.84	24.00	16.00	15.00	11.00	11.00	11.00	11.00
1	25.00	25.00	20.00	18.00	16.00	9.00	10.00	6.00
1	15.00	22.00	15.00	17.57	12.00	9.00	8.00	6.50
1	26.00	20.00	7.00	2.00	1.00	0.00	0.00	2.00
1	22.00	20.00	12.13	8.00	6.00	3.00	2.00	3.00
1	24.00	25.00	15.00	24.00	18.00	15.19	13.00	12.32
1	22.00	18.00	17.00	6.00	2.00	2.00	0.00	1.00
1	27.00	26.00	1.00	18.00	10.00	13.00	12.00	10.00
1	22.00	20.00	27.00	13.00	9.00	8.00	4.00	5.00
1	20.00	17.00	20.00	10.00	8.89	8.49	7.02	6.79
1	22.00	22.00	12.00	−9.00	−9.00	−9.00	−9.00	−9.00
1	20.00	22.00	15.38	2.00	4.00	6.00	3.00	3.00
1	21.00	23.00	11.00	9.00	10.00	8.00	7.00	4.00
1	17.00	17.00	15.00	−9.00	−9.00	−9.00	−9.00	−9.00
1	18.00	22.00	7.00	12.00	15.00	−9.00	−9.00	−9.00
1	23.00	26.00	24.00	−9.00	−9.00	−9.00	−9.00	−9.00

0 = placebo, 1 = active, −9.00 indicates a missing values.

persisted for up to 18 months post-natally. Thirty-four of the women were randomly allocated to the active treatment: 3 months of trans-dermal 17β-oestradiol 200 μg daily alone, followed by 3 months with added cyclical dydrogeterone 10 mg daily for 12 days each month. The remaining 27 women received placebo patches and tablets according to the same regimen. The main outcome variable was a composite measure of depression recorded on two occasions before randomisation, and on six two monthly visits after randomisation. Not all of the 61 women had the depression variable recorded on all eight scheduled visits.

In Fig. 5.1, the data of all the 61 women are shown, separated into treatment groups. Lines connect the repeated observations for each woman. This simple graph makes a number of features of the data readily apparent. First, almost all the women are becoming less depressed. Second, the women who are most depressed at the beginning of the study tend to be most depressed throughout. This phenomenon is generally referred to as *tracking*. Third, there are substantial individual differences and variability appears to increase over the course of the trial.

The tracking phenomenon can be seen rather more clearly in a plot of the standardised values of each observation, i.e., the values obtained by subtracting the relevant visit mean from the original observation and then dividing by the corresponding visit standard deviation. The resulting graph appears in Fig. 5.2.

With large numbers of observations, graphical displays of individual response profiles are of little use and investigators then commonly produce graphs showing the average profiles for each treatment group along with some indication of the variation of the observations at each time point. Fig. 5.3 shows such a plot for the oestrogen patch trial example. The general decline in depression values over time in both the active and placebo groups is apparent as is the lower level of depression scores in the former group. An alternative to this type of plot is to graph side-by-side box plots of the observations at each time point — see Fig. 5.4.

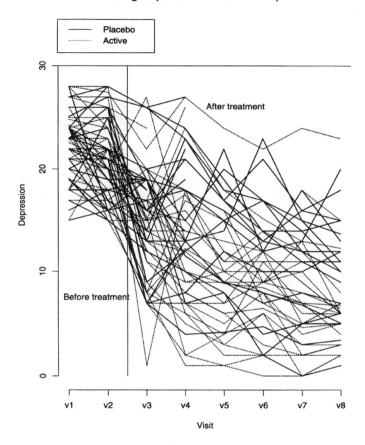

Fig. 5.1. Individual response profiles by treatment group for the oestrogen patch data.

An important aspect of the longitudinal data collected in many clinical trials is the degree of association of the repeated measurements. Finding a parsimonious model which describes the pattern of associations accurately is often a crucial part of fitting the models to be described in Chapters 6 and 7. It is frequently useful to have some graphical display to guide the search for a realistic model; one

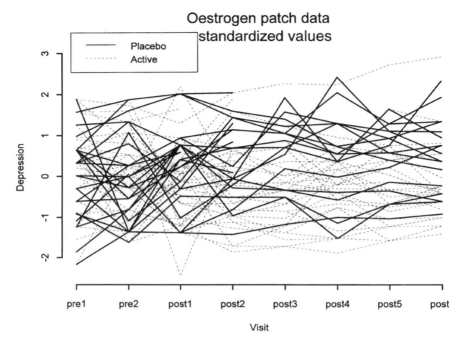

Fig. 5.2. Individual response profiles for oestrogen patch data after standardisation.

display which can be helpful is the *scatterplot matrix* in which scat-
terplots of pairs of repeated measurements are placed together in a
grid. Such a plot for the data from the trial of oestrogen patches
is shown in Fig. 5.5. We see that the degree of correlation between
the pairs of observations generally decreases as the time between
them increases.

As an illustration of what can be achieved with graphical displays
on even very large sets of data, we will use an example reported by
Zeger and Katz (1998) involving an investigation of the effects of
vitamin A supplementation on Nepali pre-school children's morbidity
and mortality. Figure 5.6 shows growth data collected in the study
from children receiving placebos. Each child was measured on up to
5 visits at four monthly intervals and the data in Fig. 5.6 consists

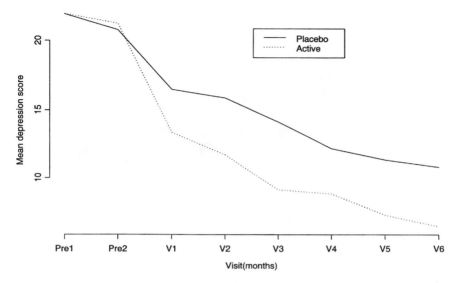

Fig. 5.3. Mean response profiles for active and placebo groups in the oestrogen patch trial.

of 11 290 observations on 2 237 children. Since here connecting the repeated measurements for *all* children would produce a completly useless graphic, the measurements of a subset of 100 children have been joined to communicate the degree of consistency across time in a child's weight as well as variation in weight among children. Half of these children were selected at random and the remaining 50 were children having average weights extreme for their age. The following characteristics of the data are apparent from Fig. 5.6.

- The average weight of the Nepali children increases by about one kilogram per month for the first six months, and then the growth rate slows dramatically to less than a quarter of the original rate.
- There is much greater variability in weight across children than across time for a given child, i.e., there is strong tracking of children's weight so that repeated observations on the same child will be highly correlated.

Boxplots for placebo

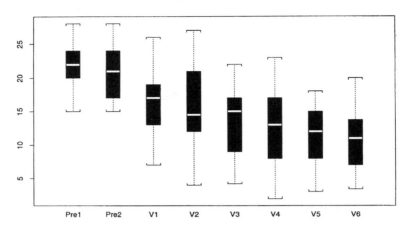

Boxplots for active

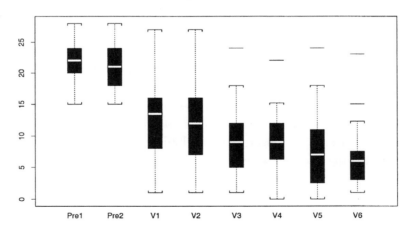

Fig. 5.4. Box-plots for data from the oestrogen patch data.

- There is some indication that the rate of growth is greater for larger children as evidenced by more positive slopes above the average curve than below.

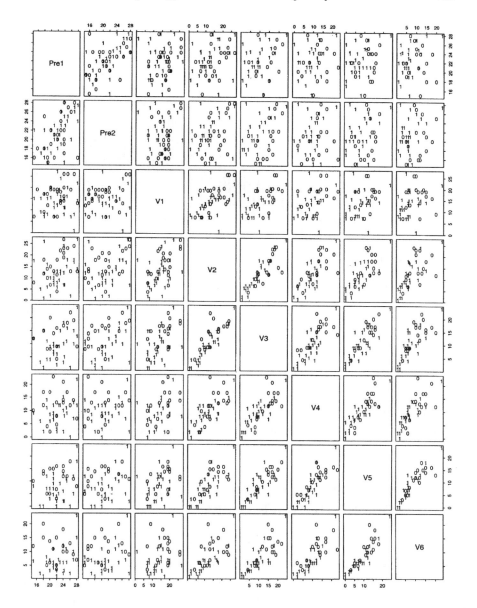

Fig. 5.5. Scatterplot matrix for the data from the oestrogen patch trial.

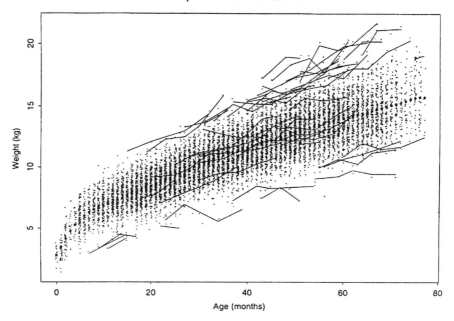

Fig. 5.6. Scatterplot of 11 290 weights on 2 337 Nepali children. Bold dots indicate a smoothing spline with 22 equivalent degrees of freedom as an estimate of the mean weigh at each age. The repeated observations for 100 children are connected — 50 chosen at random and 50 with extreme mean weights for their age (taken with permission from Zeger and Katz, 1998).

5.3. TIME-BY-TIME ANALYSIS OF LONGITUDINAL DATA

A time-by-time analysis of the longitudinal data consists of T separate analyses, one for each sub-set of data corresponding to each observation time. If only two treatment groups are being compared, each analysis consists of a t-test (or if thought necessary, its nonparametric equivalent) to assess the difference in the means (medians) of the two groups at each time point. If more than two groups are

Table 5.2. Time-by-Time Analysis of Data from Oestrogen Patch Trial.

Group		V1	V2	V3	V4	V5	V6
Placebo	Mean	16.48	15.89	14.13	12.27	11.40	10.89
	SD	5.28	6.12	4.97	5.85	4.44	4.68
	n	27	22	17	17	17	17
Active	Mean	13.37	11.74	9.13	8.83	7.31	6.59
	SD	5.56	6.57	5.47	4.67	5.74	4.73
	n	34	31	29	28	28	28
95% CI		(0.31, 5.91)	(0.59, 7.71)	(1.77, 8.23)	(0.28, 6.60)	(0.83, 7.34)	(1.40, 7.20)

involved, an analysis of variance is applied to the data at each ob-servation time (or again perhaps some suitable nonparametric alter-native). Relevant covariate information might be incorporated into each analysis.

As an illustration of this approach, Table 5.2 shows the results of applying t-tests and calculating confidence intervals for the available data at each of the six post-randomisation visits in the oestrogen patch trial. At each visit, there is a significant difference in the mean depression scores of the active and placebo groups.

Although Finney (1990) suggests that the time-by-time approach to the analysis of the longitudinal data might be quite useful if the occasions are few and the intervals between them are large, it has, in general, several serious drawbacks. One problem is that the struc-ture of the data is ignored; at no stage does this type of analysis use the information that indicates which observations are from the same individual. Consequently, the standard errors are based on between-subject variation only, and this is unlikely to lead to an analysis that is fully efficient. A further problem is that inferences made within each of the T separate analyses are not independent, nor is it clear how they should be combined. Simply assuming that the tests give *independent* information about group differences is clearly not sensible, as is demonstrated by considering what would happen if the repeated measurements were made more frequently. The number of significance tests performed would rise accordingly, but the increase in information about the difference between treatments is likely to be small.

Repeated testing also implicitly assumes that each time point is of interest in its own right; this is unlikely to be so in most applications, where the real interest will be in something more global. It is highly questionable whether the hypotheses being tested by the time-by-time approach, namely the equality of the group means at each time point, are of interest. Such an analysis does not give an overall answer to whether or not there is a treatment difference and provides no single estimate of the treatment effect.

A time-by-time analysis is not, in general, appropriate for analysing data collected over time in a clinical trial, since it simply ignores the longitudinal nature of the observations. There may, however, be some instances where the method can lead to useful results if it concentrates on exactly the right feature of the data, as shown in a non clinical trial context by Kenward (1987). Trying to find some feature of the data that characterises concisely their structure is also central to another simple, but in this case often very useful, method for the analysis of longitudinal data from clinical trials, namely the *response feature* or *summary measures* approach.

5.4. RESPONSE FEATURE ANALYSIS OF LONGITUDINAL DATA

The use of summary measures is one of the most important and straightforward approaches to the analysis of longitudinal data (at least when there are few missing values, and when the repeated measurements on each subject are made at the same time points). If the measurements made on the ith individual in the study are written as the vector $\mathbf{x}'_i = [x_{i1}, \ldots, x_{iT}]$, then a scalar-valued function f is chosen so that $s_i = f(\mathbf{x}_i)$ captures some essential feature of the response over time (see Section 5.3.1 for more details). In this way, the essentially multivariate nature of the repeated observations is reduced to a univariate one. This approach has been in use for many years, and is described in Oldham (1962), Yates (1982) and Matthews *et al.* (1990). Various aspects of response feature analysis will be considered in this section including how to incorporate covariates, how to deal with unbalanced data, and the implication for the method of having missing values. We begin, however, with perhaps the most important consideration, namely the choice of summary measure.

5.4.1. Choosing Summary Measures

To begin with, we shall assume that the response variable observed over time is continuous (or quasi-continuous) but not necessarily normally distributed. The key step to a successful response feature analysis is the choice of a relevant summary measure f. In most cases, the decision over what is a suitable measure should to be made *before* the data are collected. The chosen summary measure needs to be relevant to the particular questions of interest in the study and in the broader scientific context in which the study takes place. In some longitudinal studies, more than a single summary measure might be deemed relevant or necessary, in which case the problem of combined inference may need to be addressed. More often in practice, however, it is likely that the different measures will deal with substantially different questions so that each will have a natural interpretation in its own right.

A wide range of possible summary measures have been proposed. Those given in Table 5.3, for example, were suggested by Matthews *et al.* (1990). Frison and Pocock (1992) argue that the average response to treatment over time is often likely to be the most relevant summary statistic in treatment trials. In some cases the response on a particular visit may be chosen as the summary statistic of most interest, but this must be distinguished from the generally flawed approach which separately analyses the observations at each and every time point.

Table 5.3. Possible Summary Measures (from Matthews *et al.*, 1990).

Type of Data	Questions of Interest	Summary Measure
Peaked	Is overall value of outcome variable the same in different groups?	Overall mean (equal time intervals) or area under curve (unequal intervals)
Peaked	Is maximum (minimum) response different between groups?	Maximum (minimum) value
Peaked	Is time to maximum (minimum) response different between groups?	Time to maximum (minimum) response
Growth	Is rate of change of outcome different between groups?	Regression coefficient
Growth	Is eventual value of outcome different between groups?	Final value of outcome or difference between last and first values or percentage change between first and last values
Growth	Is response in one group delayed relative to the other?	Time to reach a particular value (e.g. a fixed percentage of baseline)

As our first example of the application of the summary measure technique, we will use the data shown in Table 5.4. These data arise from an investigation of the use of lecithin, a precursor of choline, in the treatment of Alzheimer's disease. Traditionally, it has been assumed that this condition involves an inevitable and progressive deterioration in all aspects of intellect, self-care, and personality.

Table 5.4. Data from Trial of Lecithin for the Treatment of Alzheimer's Disease.

Group	V1	V2	V3	V4	V5
1	20	19	20	20	18
1	14	15	16	9	6
1	7	5	8	8	5
1	6	10	9	10	10
1	9	7	9	5	6
1	9	10	9	11	11
1	7	3	7	6	3
1	18	20	20	23	21
1	6	10	10	13	14
1	10	15	15	15	14
1	5	9	7	3	12
1	11	11	8	10	9
1	10	2	9	3	2
1	17	12	14	15	13
1	16	15	13	7	9
1	7	10	4	10	5
1	5	0	5	0	0
1	16	7	7	6	10
1	5	6	9	5	6
1	2	1	1	2	2
1	7	11	7	5	11
1	9	16	17	10	6
1	2	5	6	7	6
1	7	3	5	5	5
1	19	13	19	17	17
1	7	5	8	8	6
2	9	11	14	11	14
2	6	7	9	12	16
2	13	18	14	20	14
2	9	10	9	8	7
2	6	7	4	5	4

Table 5.4 (*Continued*)

Group	V1	V2	V3	V4	V5
2	11	11	5	10	12
2	7	10	11	8	5
2	8	18	19	15	14
2	3	3	3	1	3
2	4	10	9	17	10
2	11	10	5	15	16
2	1	3	2	2	5
2	6	7	7	6	7
2	0	3	2	0	0
2	18	19	15	17	20
2	15	15	15	14	12
2	14	11	8	10	8
2	6	6	5	5	8
2	10	10	6	10	9
2	4	6	6	4	2
2	4	13	9	8	7
2	14	7	8	10	6

1 = placebo, 2 = lecithin

Recent work suggests that the disease involves pathological changes in the central cholinergic system, which it might be possible to remedy by long-term dietary enrichment with lecithin. In particular, the treatment might slow down or perhaps even halt the memory impairment usually associated with the condition. Patients suffering from Alzheimer's disease were randomly allocated to receive either lecithin or placebo for a six-month period. A cognitive test score giving the number of words recalled from a previously studied list was recorded at the start, at one month, at two months, at four months and at six months. As a summary measure for these data, we shall use the maximum number of words recalled on any of the five occasions of testing. (The 'maximum' was chosen on clinical advice,

Table 5.5. Results from Response Feature Approach on Data from Lecithin Trial Using Maximum Number of Words Over the Five Visits as Summary Measure.

	Placebo	Active
Mean	11.9	11.8
SD	5.0	5.2
n	26	22

95% confidence interval for difference — $(-2.9, 3.1)$

although it may have less desirable statistical properties, for example, its variance will be greater, than the mean.) The results of applying a t-test to the summary measures of each patient in the two treatment groups is given in Table 5.5. There is no evidence of any treatment effect.

As a further illustration of the response feature approach, we shall again use the data from the oestrogen patch trial given in Table 5.1. The chosen summary measure here is the mean of the post-randomisation measures. This immediately gives rise to a complication since not all the women in the trial have observations on all six occasions. The summary measure approach is often sufficiently flexible to accomodate missing values relatively simply; here, for example, we could take the mean of the *available* observations for each patient. One alternative would be to use only the women with observations on all six post-randomisation occasions and another possibility would be to use the last recorded value for a woman for all the missing values, the so-called *last observation carried forward* (LOCF) approach. (Missing values might also be imputed by, for example, substituting relevant mean values of using some more complex procedure.) The results obtained from using each approach are shown in Table 5.6. In this case, the three confidence intervals for the treatment difference are very similar. In most cases when using the response feature approach, however, particularly when the proportion of missing observations is small, using the available

Table 5.6. Results of Using Summary Measure Procedure with Mean Depression Score as Summary Measure in Oestrogen Patch Data with Various Approaches to Dealing with the Missing Values.

(1) *Mean of usable values*

	Placebo	Active
mean	14.76	10.55
sd	4.56	5.36
n	27	34

95% confidence interval for difference — $(1.61, 6.79)$

(2) *Complete cases*

	Placebo	Active
mean	13.38	9.30
sd	4.28	4.57
n	17	28

95% confidence interval for difference — $(1.33, 6.82)$

(3) *Last observation carried forward*

	Placebo	Active
mean	14.95	10.66
sd	4.66	5.56
n	27	34

95% confidence interval for difference — $(1.62, 6.96)$

observations to calculate the summary measure is recommended although with accompanying caveats about two potential problems:

- If the summary measure s_i are based on observations $\mathbf{x}_i$ made at considerably different sets of time points (either by design or because of the occurrence of missing values), then the standard t-test or analysis of variance assumption of a common variance for all observations can no longer be true. Means based on different numbers of observations, regression slopes based on differently located observations, and maxima within sets of observations of different sizes, will not share common distributions. The likely importance and impact of this problem will need to be judged in each particular application. (Matthews, 1993, describes a refinement of the response feature approach which goes some way to dealing with the problem of observations at irregular time points. The central idea of Matthew's proposal is to introduce some form of weighting into the estimation of the treatment difference.)

- The *type* of missing value (see Chapter 2) has implications for the suitability of the summary measure approach. When the observations are missing completely at random, calculating the chosen summary measure from the available observations is a valid and acceptable procedure as is using only complete cases, although the latter will be less efficient particularly if there, is a considerable proportion of intended observations that are missing. But if the missing values are thought to be other than MCAR, response feature analysis may be seriously misleading. If, for example, interest focuses on the maximum depression score over time, and some adverse effect of severe depression stops them from being observed (the patient cannot attend the clinic perhaps), then simply using the maximum of the observations that were obtained would clearly not be acceptable.

Imputing missing values before calculating summary measures is also not without its problems. Using the last observation carried forward (LOCF) method in which each missing value is substituted by the subject's last available assessment of the same type is often used, particularly in the pharmaceutical industry. But the method appears to have little in its favour except that it records what has been achievable with a particular patient. The procedure involves, however, highly unlikely assumptions, for example, that the expected value of the (unobserved) post dropout responses remain at their last recorded value.

Imputation methods need to be carefully chosen to avoid biased estimates from filled-in data. Also, imputation invents data, and analysing filled-in data as if they were complete leads to overstatement of precision, i.e., standard errors are underestimated, stated p-values of tests are too small, and confidence intervals do not cover the true parameter at the stated rate. More will be said about imputation in other contexts in Chapters 6 and 7.

Although the simple summary measures listed in Table 5.3 are the ones most likely to be commonly used, Gornbein *et al.* (1992) and Diggle *et al.* (1994) urge a more imaginative use of the summary measure approach, with the fitting of scientifically interpretable *nonlinear* models to the observations collected on each individual and the use of derived parameter stimates as the summary measures for analysis. An example given by Gornbein *et al.* (1992) involves a study to compare the relationship between parathyroid hormone (PTH) and serum ionized calcium (ICa) in normal teenagers versus teenagers undergoing dialysis for end stage renal disease. As ICa levels are artificially lowered or raised in the serum, the parathyroid gland senses the change and responds by altering the production of PTH. Increased levels of PTH cause more calcium to be released from the bones. Decreased levels result in more calcium absorption by the bones. In this way, the body attempts to restore the serum ICa to a 'setpoint' level. Based on this biological model, the investigators expected to see a sigmoid relationship between ICa and PTH.

The data were incomplete for some subjects as the PTH samples taken at a given ICa level were sometimes contaminated, lost or spoiled. In addition, the same ICa levels were not used for all subjects. The following normal sigmoid model was fitted to each partcipant's repeated observations:

$$y = \beta_0 + \beta_1/[1 + (x/\beta_2)^{\exp(\beta_3)}] + \epsilon, \epsilon \sim N(0, \sigma^2) \qquad (5.1)$$

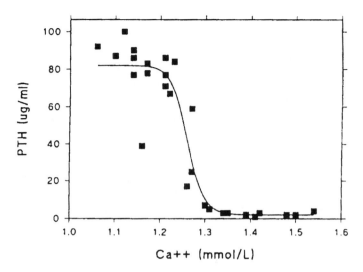

Fig. 5.7. Observations and fitted curve for one subject's data in study of parathyroid hormone (taken with permission from Gornbein *et al.*, 1992).

(The observation and fitted curve for one subject are shown in Fig. 5.7.)

Each subject's original data are now summarised by the four parameters $\beta_0, \beta_1, \beta_2$ and β_3. Normal volunteers can be compared to diseased subjects by comparing these four parameters, rather than by comparing mean profiles. (Since there are four parameters, a multivariate test such as Hotelling's T^2 might be needed.) As these parameters have a physical meaning, this sort of comparison is generally easier to interpret than one involving mean profiles.

5.4.2. Incorporating Pre-Randomisation, Baseline Measures into the Response Feature Approach

Baseline measurements of the outcome variable, if available, can be used in association with the response feature method in a number of ways. Frisson and Pocock (1992), for example, suggest three possibilities when the average response over time is the chosen summary measure:

- POST — an analysis that ignores the pre-randomisation values available and analyses only the mean of each subject's post-randomisation responses;
- CHANGE — an analysis that uses the differences between the means of each subject's post- and pre-randomisation responses;
- ANCOVA — here between subject variation in baseline measurements is taken into account by using the mean of the baseline values for each subject as a covariate in a linear model for the comparison of post-randomisation means.

The mathematical details of each approach in the simplest case of a single baseline measure and a single post-randomisation measure are shown in Table 5.7. It is clear that the estimation of the treatment effect in each case differ in how the observed difference at outcome is adjusted for the baseline difference. POST, for example, relies on the fact that in a randomised trial, in the absence of a difference between treatments, the expected value of the mean difference at outcome is zero. Hence, the factor by which the observed outcome needs correcting in order to judge the treatment effect, is also zero.

The CHANGE approach corresponds to the assumption that the difference at outcome, in the absence of a treatment effect, is expected to be equal to the difference in the means of the baselines. In the context of many clinical trials, however, this assumption may be false as is well documented by a variety of authors, e.g., Chuang-Stein and Tong (1997), Chuang-Stein (1993) and Senn (1994a, 1994b). The difficulty primarily involves the *regression to the mean*, phenomenon. This refers to the process that occurs as transient components of an initial score are dissipated over time. Selection of high scoring individuals for entry into a trial necessarily also selects for individuals with high values of any transient component that might contribute to that score. Remeasurement during the trial will tend to show

Table 5.7. POST, CHANGE and ANCOVA compared.

- We will consider a randomised parallel groups clinical trial for which baseline and final values are available for each member of the control and treatment groups.
- Measurements on members of the treatment group are represented by X_{ti} (baselines) and Y_{ti} (outcomes), $i = 1, \ldots, n_t$. Similarly, measurements in the control group are represented by X_{ci} and Y_{ci}, $i = 1, \ldots, n_c$.
- Suppose that the covariance matrix, $\Sigma_{X,Y}$, in the two groups is identical and given by:

$$\Sigma_{X,Y} = \begin{pmatrix} \sigma_X^2 & \rho\sigma_X\sigma_Y \\ \rho\sigma_X\sigma_Y & \sigma_Y^2 \end{pmatrix}$$

- When POST is the method of analysis, the effect of treatment is estimated as $\hat{\tau}_{\text{raw}} = \bar{Y}_t - \bar{Y}_c$ with variance var $(\hat{\tau}_{\text{raw}}) = q\sigma_Y^2$ where $q = \frac{1}{n_t} + \frac{1}{n_c}$.
- When CHANGE is used, the effect of treatment is estimated as $\tau_{\text{change}} = (\bar{Y}_t - \bar{X}_t) - (\bar{Y}_c - \bar{X}_c) = (\bar{Y}_t - \bar{Y}_c) - (\bar{X}_t - \bar{X}_c)$ with variance var$(\hat{\tau}_{\text{change}}) = q(\sigma_Y^2 + \sigma_X^2 - 2\rho\sigma_X\sigma_Y)$.
- A more general estimator of the treatment effect is given by $\hat{\tau}_\beta = (\bar{Y}_t - \bar{Y}_c) - \beta(\bar{X}_t - \bar{X}_c)$ which has variance var$(\hat{\tau}_\beta) = q[(\beta\sigma_X - \rho\sigma_Y)^2 + (1 - \rho^2)\sigma_Y^2]$. ANCOVA corresponds to choosing a suitable value for β, namely $\beta' = \rho\sigma_Y/\sigma_X$.
- The raw-outcomes and change-score estimator are special forms of the general estimator with $\beta = 0$ and $\beta = 1$.
- The three methods POST, CHANGE and ANCOVA can now be seen merely as ways of adjusting the observed difference at outcome using the baseline difference.
- POST relies on the fact that in a randomised trial, in the absence of a treatment effect, the expected value of the mean difference at outcome is zero. Hence the factor by which the observed outcome needs correcting, in order to judge the treatment effect, is also zero.
- CHANGE corresponds to the assumption that the difference at outcome, in the absence of a treatment effect, is expected to be the diffference in the means of the baselines. This assumption is, in fact, false (see, for example, Senn, 1994).
- ANCOVA allows for a more general system of predicting what the outcome difference would have been in the absence of any treatment effect as a function of the mean difference at baseline

(The above is an abbreviated version of Senn, 1998, from where a more detailed account is available.)

a declining mean value for such groups. Consequently, groups that initially differ through the existence of transient phenomena such as some forms of measurement error, will show a tendency to have converged on remeasurement. Randomisation ensures only that treatment groups are similar only in terms of expected values and so may actually differ not just in transient phenomena but also in more permanent components of the observed scores. Thus, while the dissipation of transient components may bring about regression to the mean phenomena such as those previously described, the extent of regression and the mean value to which the separate groups are regressing need not be expected to be the same. Analysis of covariance (ANCOVA) allows for such differences. The use of ANCOVA allows for some more general system of predicting what the outcome difference would have been in the absence of any treatment effect, as a function of the mean difference at baseline.

Frison and Pocock (1992) compare the three approaches when different numbers of pre-randomisation measurements are available. With a single baseline measure of the outcome variable, they show that analysis of covariance is more powerful than both analysis of change scores and analysis of post-randomisation means only, except when the correlations between the repeated measurements are small. Using the mean of several pre-randomisation measures (if available), makes the analysis of covariance even more efficient if there are substantial correlations between the repeated observations.

The differences between the three approaches can be illustrated by comparing power curves calculated using the results given in Frison and Pocock (1992). Figures 5.8, 5.9 and 5.10 show some examples for the situation with two treatment groups, two pre-randomisation values and six post-randomisation observations and varying degrees of association between the repeated observations (the correlations between pairs of repeated measurements are assumed equal in the calculation of these power curves). From these curves, it can be seen that the sample size needed to achieve a particular power for detecting a standardised treatment difference of 0.5 is always *lower* with

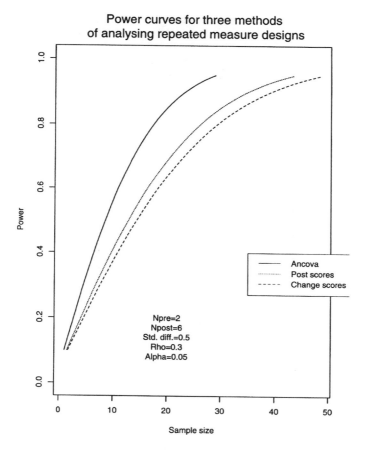

Fig. 5.8. Power curves for POST, CHANGE and ANCOVA.

analysis of covariance, and in some cases, substantially lower. As the correlation between the repeated observations increases, CHANGE approaches ANCOVA in power, with both being considerably better than POST. With a low correlation of 0.2, however, CHANGE does less well than simply dealing with post-randomisation values only. (When the correlation is zero, ANCOVA and POST are essentially equivalent.)

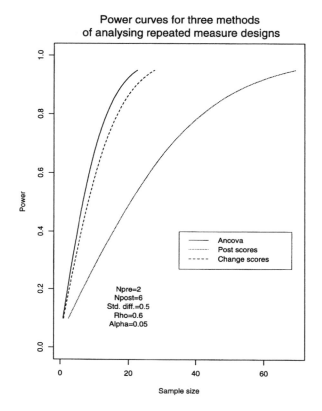

Fig. 5.9. Power curves for POST, CHANGE and ANCOVA.

The results of applying each of POST, CHANGE and ANCOVA to the oestrogen patch example, using the mean of available post-randomisation observation as the response and the mean of available pre-randomisation measures as baseline, are shown in Table 5.8. Here, all three approaches indicate a substantial treatment effect.

5.4.3. Response Feature Analysis when the Response Variable is Binary

Table 5.9 shows the data collected in a clinical trial comparing two treatments for a respiratory illness (Davis, 1991). In each of the two

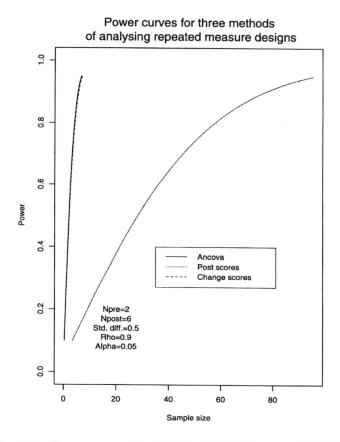

Fig. 5.10. Power curves for POST, CHANGE and ANCOVA.

centres, eligible patients were randomly assigned to active treatment or placebo. During treatment, the respiratory status (categorised as 0 = poor, 1 = good) was determined at four visits. There were 111 patients (54 active, 57 placebo) with no missing data for responses or covariates. Some detailed analyses of these data will be described in Chapter 7, but here we shall consider how the response feature approach could be used. We might, of course, simply ignore the binary nature of the response variable and compare the 'mean' responses over time in the two treatment groups by a *t*-test.

Table 5.8. Application of POST, CHANGE and ANCOVA to Mean Depression Scores used as Response and Covariate (means of usable values).

(1) POST

95% confidence interval for difference — $(1.61, 6.79)$
(Details given in Table 5.6).

(2) CHANGE

	Placebo	Active
mean	−6.51	−11.07
sd	4.38	5.49
n	27	34

95% confidence interval for difference — $(1.97, 7.16)$

(3) ANCOVA

Placebo Adjusted Mean	Active Adjusted Mean
14.85	10.47

Mean square from analysis of covariance is 23.29 based on 58 degrees of freedom.
95% confidence interval for difference — $(1.89, 6.87)$

Since the mean in this case is the proportion (p) of visits at which a patient's respiratory status was good, we could consider performing the test after taking some appropriate transformation, for example, $\arcsin(p)$ or $\arcsin(\sqrt{p})$. All such tests indicate that there is a substantial difference between the two treatments. A linear regression of the arcsin transformed proportion of positive responses over the four post-baseline measurement occasions might be used to assess the effects of the baseline measurement, age, sex and centre. The results are shown in Table 5.10

A more satisfactory analysis can be achieved by using the GLM approach described in the previous chapter. A standard logistic

Table 5.9. Respiratory Disorder Data.

Patient	Treat.	Sex	Age	BL	V1	V2	V3	V4
Centre 1								
1	P	M	46	0	0	0	0	0
2	P	M	28	0	0	0	0	0
3	A	M	23	1	1	1	1	1
4	P	M	44	1	1	1	1	0
5	P	F	13	1	1	1	1	1
6	A	M	34	0	0	0	0	0
7	P	M	43	0	1	0	1	1
8	A	M	28	0	0	0	0	0
9	A	M	31	1	1	1	1	1
10	P	M	37	1	0	1	1	0
11	A	M	30	1	1	1	1	1
12	A	M	14	0	1	1	1	0
13	P	M	23	1	1	0	0	0
14	P	M	30	0	0	0	0	0
15	P	M	20	1	1	1	1	1
16	A	M	22	0	0	0	0	1
17	P	M	25	0	0	0	0	0
18	A	F	47	0	0	1	1	1
19	P	F	31	0	0	0	0	0
20	A	M	20	1	1	0	1	0
21	A	M	26	0	1	0	1	0
22	A	M	46	1	1	1	1	1
23	A	M	32	1	1	1	1	1
24	A	M	48	0	1	0	0	0
25	P	F	35	0	0	0	0	0
26	A	M	26	0	0	0	0	0
27	P	M	23	1	1	0	1	1
28	P	F	36	0	1	1	0	0
29	P	M	19	0	1	1	0	0
30	A	M	28	0	0	0	0	0
31	P	M	37	0	0	0	0	0

Table 5.9 (*Continued*)

Patient	Treat.	Sex	Age	BL	V1	V2	V3	V4
32	A	M	23	0	1	1	1	1
33	A	M	30	1	1	1	1	0
34	P	M	15	0	0	1	1	0
35	A	M	26	0	0	0	1	0
36	P	F	45	0	0	0	0	0
37	A	M	31	0	0	1	0	0
38	A	M	50	0	0	0	0	0
39	P	M	28	0	0	0	0	0
40	P	M	26	0	0	0	0	0
41	P	M	14	0	0	0	0	1
42	A	M	31	0	0	1	0	0
43	P	M	13	1	1	1	1	1
44	P	M	27	0	0	0	0	0
45	P	M	26	0	1	0	1	1
46	P	M	49	0	0	0	0	0
47	P	M	63	0	0	0	0	0
48	A	M	57	1	1	1	1	1
49	P	M	27	1	1	1	1	1
50	A	M	22	0	0	1	1	1
51	A	M	15	0	0	1	1	1
52	P	M	43	0	0	0	1	0
53	A	F	32	0	0	0	1	0
54	A	M	11	1	1	1	1	0
55	P	M	24	1	1	1	1	1
56	A	M	25	0	1	1	0	1
Centre 2								
1	P	F	39	0	0	0	0	0
2	A	M	25	0	0	1	1	1
3	A	M	58	1	1	1	1	1
4	P	F	51	1	1	0	1	1
5	P	F	32	1	0	0	1	1
6	P	M	45	1	1	0	0	0

Table 5.9 (*Continued*)

Patient	Treat.	Sex	Age	BL	V1	V2	V3	V4
7	P	F	44	1	1	1	1	1
8	P	F	48	0	0	0	0	0
9	A	M	26	0	1	1	1	1
10	A	M	14	0	1	1	1	1
11	P	F	48	0	0	0	0	0
12	A	M	13	1	1	1	1	1
13	P	M	20	0	1	1	1	1
14	A	M	37	1	1	0	0	1
15	A	M	25	1	1	1	1	1
16	A	M	20	0	0	0	0	0
17	P	F	58	0	1	0	0	0
18	P	M	38	1	1	0	0	0
19	A	M	55	1	1	1	1	1
20	A	M	24	1	1	1	1	1
21	P	F	36	1	1	0	0	1
22	P	M	36	0	1	1	1	1
23	A	F	60	1	1	1	1	1
24	P	M	15	1	0	0	1	1
25	A	M	25	1	1	1	1	0
26	A	M	35	1	1	1	1	1
27	A	M	19	1	1	0	1	1
28	P	F	31	1	1	1	1	1
29	A	M	21	1	1	1	1	1
30	A	F	37	0	1	1	1	1
31	P	M	52	0	1	1	1	1
32	A	M	55	0	0	1	1	0
33	P	M	19	1	0	0	1	1
34	P	M	20	1	0	1	1	1
35	P	M	42	1	0	0	0	0
36	A	M	41	1	1	1	1	1
37	A	M	52	0	0	0	0	0
38	P	F	47	0	1	1	0	1

Table 5.9 (*Continued*)

Patient	Treat.	Sex	Age	BL	V1	V2	V3	V4
39	P	M	11	1	1	1	1	1
40	P	M	14	0	0	0	1	0
41	P	M	15	1	1	1	1	1
42	P	M	66	1	1	1	1	1
43	A	M	34	0	1	1	0	1
44	P	M	43	0	0	0	0	0
45	P	M	33	1	1	1	0	0
46	P	M	48	1	1	0	0	0
47	A	M	20	0	1	1	1	1
48	P	F	39	1	0	1	0	0
49	A	M	28	0	1	0	0	0
50	P	F	38	0	0	0	0	0
51	A	M	43	1	1	1	1	0
52	A	F	39	0	1	1	1	1
53	A	M	68	0	1	1	1	1
54	A	F	63	1	1	1	1	1
55	A	M	31	1	1	1	1	1

Treatment: P = placebo, A = active,
Gender: M = male, F = female,
Response: 0 = respiratory status poor, 1 = respiratory status good.

Table 5.10. Results from a Linear Regression of the Arcsin Transformed Response of Positive Responses over the Four Post-baseline Measurement Occasions for the Respiratory Data in Table 5.9.

Covariate	Estimate	SE	p
Treatment	0.377	0.101	< 0.001
Baseline	0.580	0.103	< 0.001
Age/100	−0.402	0.386	0.3
Sex	0.039	0.133	0.8
Centre	0.205	0.107	0.06

Table 5.11. Results from a GLM for a Logit Model Allowing for Overdispersion for the Respiratory Data in Table 5.9.

Covariate	Estimate Odds Ratio	SE	p
Treatment	3.544	1.208	< 0.001
Baseline	6.333	2.197	< 0.001
Age/100	0.153	0.196	0.1
Sex	1.147	0.488	0.7
Centre	1.915	0.661	0.06

regression model might be applied but since the number of occasions on which infection was present out of the 4 visits made by each participant is unlikely to be binomially distributed (the observations are likely to be correlated rather than independent), we need to allow for possible overdispersion. This is relatively straightforward using the quasilikelihood procedure of Wedderburn (1974) to fit a GLM for overdispersed binomial data with variance function $\phi\mu(1-\mu)/4$, where ϕ is estimated as described in the previous chapter.

Fitting a model with logistic link and with treatment, sex, age and baseline respiratory status as the main effects gives the results shown in Table 5.11. The estimated value of the scale parameter, 2.10, is substantially above one confirming the presence of overdispersion. The estimated odds ratio for the effect of treatment is 3.54, with a 95% confidence interval of $(1.82, 6.91)$.

The p-values from the linear regression in Table 5.10 and the logistic regression in Table 5.11 are comparable, but the estimates from the logit model are on a more natural scale. There is no relatively straightforward interpretation of the estimates from the model fitted to the arcsin transformed responses, although calculation of an odds-ratio at the mean value of the sample covariates could be attempted.

5.5. SUMMARY

The methods described in this chapter provide for the exploration and simple analysis of longitudinal data collected in the course of a clinical trial. The graphical methods can provide insights into both potentially interesting patterns of response over time and the structure of any treatment differences. In addition, they can indicate possible outlying observations that may need special attention. The response feature approach to analysis has the distinct advantage that it is straightforward, can be tailored to consider aspects of the data thought to be particularly relevant, and produces results which are relatively simple to understand. The method can accomodate data containing missing values without difficulty, although it might be misleading if the observations are anything other than missing completely at random.

CHAPTER 6

Multivariate Normal Regression Models for Longitudinal Data from Clinical Trials

6.1. INTRODUCTION

It cannot be overemphasised that statistical analyses of clinical trials should be no more complex than necessary. So even when repeated measures data have been collected it is not always essential to apply a formal repeated measures analysis. We have already described analyses of individual summary measures such as individual mean response scores and proportions that may often not only be statistically and scientifically adequate for the testing of simple treatment differences, but can also be more persuasive and easier to communicate than some of the more ambitious analyses that we now turn to. Nonetheless, a typical trial does not take place in a scientific vacuum in which a simple treatment difference is the only question of interest. It is more usual that, in addition to being used as the basis of formal evidence for efficacy or equivalence, even a phase III trial will gather data that may be informative as to the mode of action of the treatment, dose-response relationship, response heterogeneity, side effects and so on. In addition, attrition and variation in compliance may need to be more carefully examined than can be done within, for example, a simple summary statistics approach.

In this chapter, models suitable for analysing longitudinal data from clinical trials where the response variable can be assumed to have a conditionally normal distribution will be described. Models suitable for non normal responses will be the subject of Chapter 7.

6.2. SOME GENERAL COMMENTS ABOUT MODELS FOR LONGITUDINAL DATA

Diggle (1988) lists a number of desirable features for a general method to analyse data from studies in which outcome variables are measured at several time points. These include the following:

- the specification of the mean response profile needs to be sufficiently flexible to reflect both time trends within each treatment group and differences in these time trends between treatments. Examples of the type of mean response profiles that may need to be modelled are shown in Fig. 6.1;
- the specification of the pattern of correlations or covariances of the repeated measurements needs to be flexible, but economical;
- the method of analysis should accommodate virtually arbitrary patterns of irregularly spaced time sequences within individuals.

Although in many applications the parameters defining the covariance structure of the observations will not be of direct interest (they are often regarded as so-called *nuisance parameters*), Diggle (1988) suggests that overparametrisation will lead to inefficient estimation and potentially poor assessment of standard errors for estimates of the mean response profiles, whereas too restrictive a specification may also invalidate inferences about the mean response profiles when the assumed covariance structure does not hold.

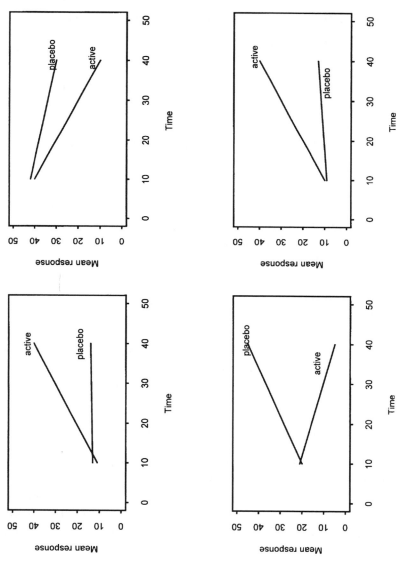

Fig. 6.1. Some examples of possible mean response profiles in longitudinal data.

In many examples, the model for the covariances and variances of the repeated measures will need to allow for *non-stationarity*, with changes (most often increases) in variances across time being particularly common. The effect of misspecifying the covariance structure when analysing longitudinal data is investigated in Rabe-Hesketh and Everitt, 1999.

In this chapter, we shall consider the likelihood methods for estimating parameters and their standard errors in very general regression-type models for longitudinal data.

Some of the advantages of using a likelihood approach are as follows:

- maximum likelihood estimates are principled in that they have known statistical properties (consistency, large sample efficiency) under the assumed model, which can be clearly specified and subjected to model criticism;
- maximum likelihood estimation does not require a rectangular data matrix and hence deals directly with the problem of unbalanced data;
- estimates are asymptotically efficient under the assumed model;
- standard errors of parameter estimates based on the observed and/or expected information matrix are available and these automatically take into account the fact that the data are incomplete.

Two disadvantages of the likelihood approach are:

- maximum likelihood estimation requires the specification of a full statistical model for the data and results may be vulnerable to departures from model assumptions (though use of the heteroscedastic consistent 'sandwich' estimator of the parameter variances introduced in Chapter 4 provides some scope for relaxing assumptions);
- maximum likelihood inferences are based on large sample theory and hence may be unsuitable for small data sets.

The details of maximum likelihood estimation of the parameters in regression models for longitudinal data will be described in Section 6.4. Before this, however, the implications for this approach of missing values due to patients dropping-out of the study need to be considered.

6.3. MISSING VALUES AND LIKELIHOOD-BASED INFERENCE FOR LONGITUDINAL DATA

In Chapter 3 a taxonomy of missing values occurring in longitudinal data was introduced. The essential distinctions drawn between missing values were:

- MCAR — *missing completely at random*, the drop-out process is independent of both the observed and missing values;
- MAR — *missing at random* the drop-out process is independent of the missing values;
- *Informative* — the drop-out process is dependent on the missing values.

For likelihood-based inference, the critical distinction is between MCAR and MAR (often referred to collectively as *ignorable*) and informative dropout since in the former case the log-likelihood function is separable into two terms, one involving the missing-data mechanism given the observed values and one only involving the observed values. The first of these contains no information about the distribution of observed values and can therefore be ignored for the purpose of making inferences about these values. (Mathematical details are given in Table 6.1.) It is important to make clear, however, that it is the missing-data mechanism that is ignorable, *not* the individuals with missing values. This is not a trivial point because one of the most common methods of analysing unbalanced longitudinal data remains using either analysis of variance or multivariate analysis of variance (see comments in Section 6.6) on complete cases.

Table 6.1. Separability of Likelihood for Non-informative Missing Values.

- Let the complete set of measurements $\mathbf{Y}^*$ be partioned into $\mathbf{Y}^* = [\mathbf{Y}^{(o)}, \mathbf{Y}^{(m)}]$, with $\mathbf{Y}^{(o)}$ representing the observed measurements and $\mathbf{Y}^{(m)}$ the missing measurements.

- Let $\mathbf{R}$ represent a set of indicator random variables denoting which elements of $\mathbf{Y}^*$ are observed and which are missing.

- Let $f(\mathbf{y}^{(o)}, \mathbf{y}^{(m)}, \mathbf{r})$ represent the joint probability density function of $(\mathbf{Y}^{(o)}, \mathbf{Y}^{(m)}, \mathbf{R})$.

- This density function can be written as:

$$f(\mathbf{y}^{(o)}, \mathbf{y}^{(m)}, \mathbf{r}) = f(\mathbf{y}^{(o)}, \mathbf{y}^{(m)}) f(\mathbf{r}|\mathbf{y}^{(o)}, \mathbf{y}^{(m)})$$

- For a likelihood-based analysis, we need the joint pdf of the observable random variables $(\mathbf{Y}^{(o)}, \mathbf{R})$, which is obtained by integrating the above to give:

$$f(\mathbf{y}^{(o)}, \mathbf{r}) = \int f(\mathbf{y}^{(o)}, \mathbf{y}^{(m)}) f(\mathbf{r}|\mathbf{y}^{(o)}, \mathbf{y}^{(m)}) d\mathbf{y}^{(m)}$$

- If the missing value mechanism is non informative, $f(\mathbf{r}|\mathbf{y}^{(o)}, \mathbf{y}^{(m)})$ does not depend on $\mathbf{y}^{(m)}$ and the above becomes:

$$
\begin{aligned}
f(\mathbf{y}^{(o)}, \mathbf{r}) &= f(\mathbf{r}|\mathbf{y}^{(o)}) \int f(\mathbf{y}^{(o)}, \mathbf{y}^{(m)}) d\mathbf{y}^{(m)} \\
&= f(\mathbf{r}|\mathbf{y}^{(o)}) f(\mathbf{y}^{(o)})
\end{aligned}
$$

- Taking logs of this expression gives:

$$L = \log f(\mathbf{r}|\mathbf{y}^{(o)}) + \log f(\mathbf{y}^{(o)})$$

- L can be maximised by separate maximisation of the two terms on the right hand side. Since the first term contains no information about the distribution of $\mathbf{Y}^{(o)}$, we can ignore it for the purposes of making inferences about $\mathbf{Y}^{(o)}$.

(The account above is taken from Diggle *et al*, 1994.)

At best (when the missing values are MCAR) such an approach is inefficient since it leaves out observations which could legitimately be used in the analysis; at worst (when the observations are MAR or informative) it may lead to erroneous inferences. The likelihood method to be described in the next section depends only on the weaker assumption that the missing values are MAR. (The difficult problems of distinguishing between random and informative missing values and of analysing data containing the latter will be dealt with in Section 6.7.)

6.4.   MAXIMUM LIKELIHOOD ESTIMATION ASSUMING NORMALITY

Following Schluchter (1988), the essence of the likelihood approach for longitudinal data possibly containing missing values is as follows:

Let $\mathbf{y}_i^*$ denote the hypothetical $T \times 1$ complete-data vector for subject i. Let $\mathbf{y}_i' = [y_{i1}, \ldots, y_{in_i}]$ be the $n_i \times 1$ vector of measurements actually present for subject $i, i = 1, 2, \ldots, n$. (We assume that measurements for subject i are made at times $t_{i1}, t_{i2}, \ldots, t_{in_i}$, i.e., we do not assume a common set of times for all subjects.) The y_{ij} are assumed to be realisations of random variables Y_{ij} which follow the regression model;

$$\mathbf{Y}_i = \mathbf{X}_i \boldsymbol{\beta} + \boldsymbol{\epsilon}_i \qquad (6.1)$$

for $i = 1, \ldots, n$, where $\mathbf{X}_i$ is a $n_i \times p$ design matrix, $\boldsymbol{\beta}$ is a $p \times 1$ vector of unknown regression coefficients. We assume that the conditional distribution of the $\mathbf{Y}_i$ given the explanatory variables is multivariate normal, i.e., that the n_i independent residual or 'error' terms in $\boldsymbol{\epsilon}_i$ have a multivariate normal distribution with zero mean vector, and covariance matrix $\boldsymbol{\Sigma}_i$. The latter is assumed to be a submatrix of a $T \times T$ matrix, $\boldsymbol{\Sigma}$, the elements of which are known functions of q unknown covariance parameters, $\boldsymbol{\theta}$, i.e., $\boldsymbol{\Sigma} = \boldsymbol{\Sigma}(\boldsymbol{\theta})$. This model will hold if the hypothetical complete-data, $\mathbf{Y}_i^*$ can be written as:

$$\mathbf{Y}_i^* = \mathbf{X}_i^* \boldsymbol{\beta} + \boldsymbol{\epsilon}_i^* \tag{6.2}$$

where $\mathbf{Y}_i, \mathbf{X}_i$ and $\boldsymbol{\epsilon}_i$ are obtained by deleting rows from $\mathbf{Y}_i^*, \mathbf{X}_i^*$ and $\boldsymbol{\epsilon}_i^*$, respectively.

Columns of each design matrix correspond to terms in the model under consideration. The first column of each $\mathbf{X}_i$, for example, is a one-vector corresponding to the intercept term; other columns may correspond to dummy variables for grouping (between-subjects, usually treatment) factors, and others to fixed and/or time varying covariates.

Maximum likelihood estimates of $\boldsymbol{\beta}$ and $\boldsymbol{\theta}$ can be found by maximizing the log-likelihood $L(\boldsymbol{\theta}, \boldsymbol{\beta})$ given by:

$$\begin{aligned}
L(\boldsymbol{\theta}, \boldsymbol{\beta}) \quad = \quad & -\frac{1}{2} \Bigg[\sum_{i=1}^{n} n_i \log(2\pi) + \sum_{i=1}^{n} \log |\boldsymbol{\Sigma}_i(\boldsymbol{\theta})| \\
& + \sum_{i=1}^{n} (\mathbf{y}_i - \mathbf{X}_i \boldsymbol{\beta})' \boldsymbol{\Sigma}_i(\boldsymbol{\theta})^{-1} (\mathbf{y}_i - \mathbf{X}_i \boldsymbol{\beta}) \Bigg]
\end{aligned} \tag{6.3}$$

Numerical optimisation techniques are required to maximise L with respect to $\boldsymbol{\beta}$ and $\boldsymbol{\theta}$. The details need not, however, concern us here (they are given in Schluchter, 1988).

The likelihood approach outlined above is implemented in a number of software packages, e.g., BMDP5V and SAS PROC MIXED (see Appendix), and such software enables the method to be applied routinely to unbalanced longitudinal data from clinical trials.

Likelihood analyses of data that do not suffer from missing values are often (but by no means universally) robust to the use of an incorrect model for the data. But with incomplete data such analyses are likely to be more sensitive to model misspecification since implicitly the data model is used to 'fill-in' for the missing values. So although valid likelihood inferences can be obtained when the data contain non-informative missing values, the validity may depend heavily upon using the correct model for the data. Consequently, examining residuals and other diagnostics for detecting model misspecification after fitting the proposed model becomes of even greater importance than usual.

A standard maximum likelihood approach as described above is known to produce *biased* estimators of the covariance parameters. In many cases this problem is unlikely to be severe, but where it *is* of concern the method of *restricted maximum likelihood* or REML estimation, introduced originally by Patterson and Thompson (1971), might be used. The details of REML estimation are given in Diggle *et al.* (1994). Often the two estimation methods will give similar results, but where they do differ substantially, those obtained from REML are generally preferred.

6.5. NUMERICAL EXAMPLES

In this section, the model outlined above will be applied to a number of examples, beginning with the trial of oestrogen patches for the treatment of post-natal depression described in Chapter 5.

6.5.1. Oestrogen Patches in the Treatment of Post-Natal Depression

Our first analysis of these data will involve the unrealistic assumption that the repeated observations are independent. Under this assumption, the model described in Section 6.3 is then simply that of multiple regression. The graphical displays of these data given in Chapter 5 suggest that there is a general decline in depression scores over time and a difference in treatment level. Additionally, there is some indication that the depression scores are beginning to 'level-off' by the end of the 12 months of the trial. This suggests considering treatment group as a covariate, and including linear and perhaps quadratic effects for time. In addition, the strong tracking observed in the plots of standardised scores over time suggests that the pre-randomisation measures should be incorporated into the model in some way — we shall use the second of the pre-randomisation measures of depression as a further covariate. The model to be considered can be written as follows:

$$y_{ijk} = \beta_0 + \beta_1 \, group + \beta_2 \, pre2 + \beta_3 \, time + \beta_4 \, time^2 + \epsilon_{ijk} \quad (6.4)$$

where *group* is a dummy variable coding treatment received, 1 for placebo and -1 for active, *pre2* is the second pre-randomisation measure and *time* takes the values 1–6 depending on the visit involved. The residual terms ϵ_{ijk} are assumed to normally distributed with means zero and variance θ. Consequently the covariance matrix, Σ, of the repeated observations in each treatment group is assumed to be:

$$\Sigma = \theta \mathbf{I} \quad (6.5)$$

where $\mathbf{I}$ is a 6×6 identity matrix.

The results from fitting this model are shown in Table 6.2. All 61 cases contribute values to the analysis despite only 45 of the women having complete data. The effects of treatment group, the pre-randomisation measure and linear time are all highly significant.

Table 6.2. Results from Likelihood Analysis of Oestrogen Patch Data (assuming independence for the repeated observations).

Parameter	Estimate	Asymp.se	z	p-value
constant	7.087	2.057	3.446	0.0006
group	2.137	0.301	7.094	< 0.0001
linear time	−2.090	0.823	−2.539	0.011
quadratic time	0.114	0.117	0.971	0.3315
baseline	0.477	0.079	6.020	< 0.0001

Approximate 95% confidence interval for treatment effect is $2 \times 2.137 \pm 1.96 \times 2 \times 0.301 = (3.09, 5.45)$

The model has a single covariance parameter; the estimated value of this parameter is 25.370 and its estimated standard error is 2.089.

The maximised log-likelihood for the model is -895.536, and Akaike's information criterion takes the value -896.536.

The independence assumption made in the analysis reported above is clearly far from the truth as Fig. 5.5 in the previous chapter demonstrates, and so we now need to consider more realistic models that allow for the repeated observations to be correlated. We shall begin with a model that allows a particular structure, *compound symmetry*, for the covariance matrix of the repeated measurements. With this structure the covariance matrix in each treatment group is assumed to be of the form:

$$\Sigma = \begin{pmatrix} \theta_1 + \theta_2 & \theta_1 & \theta_1 & \theta_1 & \theta_1 & \theta_1 \\ \theta_1 & \theta_1 + \theta_2 & \theta_1 & \theta_1 & \theta_1 & \theta_1 \\ \theta_1 & \theta_1 & \theta_1 + \theta_2 & \theta_1 & \theta_1 & \theta_1 \\ \theta_1 & \theta_1 & \theta_1 & \theta_1 + \theta_2 & \theta_1 & \theta_1 \\ \theta_1 & \theta_1 & \theta_1 & \theta_1 & \theta_1 + \theta_2 & \theta_1 \\ \theta_1 & \theta_1 & \theta_1 & \theta_1 & \theta_1 & \theta_1 + \theta_2 \end{pmatrix} \quad (6.6)$$

i.e., a common covariance equal to θ_1 and a common variance equal to $\theta_1 + \theta_2$. (As we shall see in Section 6.5, this structure arises from assuming a simple *mixed effects model* for the data and is the basis of the usual analysis of variance approach to the analysis of longitudinal data.) The covariance matrix satisfying compound symmetry can be written more concisely as follows:

$$\Sigma = \theta_1 \mathbf{1}\mathbf{1}' + \theta_2 \mathbf{I} \quad (6.7)$$

where $\mathbf{I}$ is a 6×6 identity matrix and $\mathbf{1}$ is a vector of ones.

The results from fitting a model with the same expected value for the observations as given in Eq. (6.4), but with the compound symmetry covariance structure, are shown in Table 6.3. Both the parameter estimates and their standard errors have changed from those given in Table 6.2 although the conclusions remain largely the same. The values of the log-likelihoods and Akaike's information criterion for the independence and compound symmetry models suggest that the latter represents a great improvement.

Table 6.3. Results from Likelihood Analysis of Oestrogen Patch Data (assuming compound symmetry for the covariance structure of the repeated observations).

Parameter	Estimate	Asymp.se	z	p-value
constant	7.180	3.186	2.253	0.0242
group	1.995	0.543	3.673	0.0002
linear time	-1.828	0.560	-3.263	0.0011
quadratic time	0.087	0.079	1.099	0.2719
baseline	0.460	0.145	3.174	0.0015

An approximate 95% confidence interval for the treatment effect is $(1.86, 6.12)$.

The estimates and estimated standard errors of the model's two covariance parameters are $\hat{\theta}_1 = 11.16$ (1.029) and $\hat{\theta}_2 = 14.399$ (3.149).

The maximised log-likelihood is -831.764 and Akaike's information criterion is -833.764.

Allowing a compound symmetry structure for the correlations is clearly more satisfactory than assuming that the repeated observations are independent of one another, but it remains an unrealistic assumption for the oestrogen patch data in particular and for longitudinal data in general. Both the constant variance and constant covariance assumptions are unlikely in practice. Observations taken close together in time are likely to have greater correlation than those taken far apart. Figure 5.5 certainly suggests that this is the case for the oestrogen patch data. One way to make certain that the proposed model for the covariances is adequate is to fully parameterise Σ in the sense of considering $N = T(T+1)/2$ parameters $\theta_1, \theta_2, \ldots, \theta_N$ corresponding to the unique variances and covariances $\sigma_{11}, \sigma_{21}, \ldots, \sigma_{TT}$. Such a covariance matrix is usually referred to as *unstructured*. Fitting such a model to the oestrogen patch data gives the results shown in Table 6.4. Again the parameter estimates and their standard errors change although the conclusions remain largely the same. Comparing the values of Akaike's criterion for this model with the values corresponding to the two models considered

Table 6.4. Results from Likelihood Analysis of Oestrogen Patch Data (allowing a fully parameterised covariance structure).

Parameter	Estimate	Asymp.se	z	p-value
constant	9.330	2.868	3.253	0.0011
group	2.047	0.486	4.211	< 0.0001
linear time	−1.981	0.533	−3.718	0.0002
quadratic time	0.109	0.064	1.707	0.0879
baseline	0.364	0.129	2.820	0.0048

An approximate 95% confidence interval for the treatment effect is (2.19, 6.00).

The maximised log-likelihood is −781.343 and Akaike's information criterion is −802.343.

previously shows that the unstructured covariance structure is to be preferred.

Since a fully parameterised Σ will *always* provide a perfect description of the covariance matrix of the repeated observations, the question arises as to why not use it on all occasions? For the answer we can return to the comments of Diggle (1988) already referred to in the introduction to this chapter, namely that overparameterisation can lead to inefficient estimation and potentially poor assessment of standard errors of the parameters that characterise the treatment mean profiles, i.e., those parameters that are of most interest in the majority of applications. This is a problem which is likely to be most critical when the number of observations is small relative to the number of times at which observations are made.

When using the likelihood approach described above, the missing values for subject i are imputed as follows:

$$\hat{\mathbf{y}}_{i2} = \mathbf{X}_{12}\hat{\boldsymbol{\beta}} + \hat{\boldsymbol{\Sigma}}_{21}\hat{\boldsymbol{\Sigma}}_{11}^{-1}(\mathbf{y}_i - \mathbf{X}_i\hat{\boldsymbol{\beta}}) \tag{6.8}$$

where $\mathbf{y}_i^*$ and $\mathbf{X}_i^*$ are partitioned as follows:

$$\mathbf{y}_i^* = \begin{pmatrix} \mathbf{y}_i \\ \mathbf{y}_{i2} \end{pmatrix} \quad \text{and} \quad \mathbf{X}_i^* = \begin{pmatrix} \mathbf{X}_i \\ \mathbf{X}_{i2} \end{pmatrix} \tag{6.9}$$

with $\mathbf{y}_{i2}$ representing the missing values for this subject. The terms $\hat{\mathbf{\Sigma}}_{12}$, $\hat{\mathbf{\Sigma}}_{21}$ and $\hat{\mathbf{\Sigma}}_{11}$ are appropriate submatrices of $\mathbf{\Sigma}(\hat{\boldsymbol{\theta}})$. The estimated missing values depend on the covariance structure assumed for the repeated observations; this is illustrated in Table 6.5 which shows the imputed missing values for the oestrogen patch data under each of the covariance structures considered above.

Table 6.5. Imputed Missing Values for the Oestrogen Patch Data (under three different models for the covariance structure of the repeated observations).

Subject	No. of Missing Values	Group	Model Indep.	CS	Unstruc.
3	4	placebo	11.6	12.9	12.5
			10.3	11.7	11.2
			9.2	10.6	10.1
			8.4	9.8	9.2
8	4	placebo	17.3	22.4	22.9
			16.0	21.2	20.7
			15.0	20.1	19.5
			14.1	19.2	17.3
11	5	placebo	16.9	14.4	14.7
			15.4	13.0	13.7
			14.1	11.8	12.8
			13.1	10.7	12.0
			12.2	9.8	11.8
13	4	placebo	16.4	15.6	18.8
			15.1	14.4	17.2
			14.0	13.4	16.8
			13.2	12.5	16.0
14	4	placebo	14.0	9.6	11.9
			12.7	8.4	11.1
			11.6	7.3	10.9
			10.8	6.4	11.2

Table 6.5 (*Continued*)

Subject	No. of Missing Values	Group	Model Indep.	CS	Unstruc.
15	5	placebo	15.5	16.0	15.9
			14.0	14.6	14.3
			12.7	13.4	13.1
			11.6	12.4	12.0
			10.8	11.5	11.1
16	5	placebo	16.0	16.2	16.1
			14.4	14.8	14.6
			13.2	13.6	13.3
			12.1	12.6	12.3
			11.3	11.7	11.5
23	5	placebo	13.6	13.5	13.7
			12.1	12.1	12.4
			10.8	10.9	11.2
			9.7	9.9	10.2
			8.9	9.0	9.5
25	4	placebo	13.0	14.7	16.2
			11.7	13.5	14.5
			10.7	12.5	13.7
			9.8	11.6	12.5
27	5	placebo	14.1	16.0	15.7
			12.6	14.6	14.0
			11.3	13.4	12.6
			10.2	12.3	11.4
			9.4	11.5	10.2
42	4	active	7.37	16.1	19.5
			6.0	14.9	16.5
			5.0	13.8	15.6
			4.1	13.0	12.7
45	4	active	10.7	12.0	11.4
			9.4	10.7	10.0

Table 6.5 (*Continued*)

Subject	No. of Missing Values	Group	Model Indep.	CS	Unstruc.
			8.3	9.7	8.9
			7.5	8.8	7.8
56	5	active	11.7	11.1	11.1
			10.2	9.7	9.8
			8.9	8.5	8.7
			7.8	7.4	7.8
			7.0	6.6	7.2
59	5	active	9.3	11.8	11.4
			7.8	10.4	9.7
			6.5	9.2	8.2
			5.4	8.1	7.0
			4.6	7.3	5.8
60	3	active	8.9	8.8	11.5
			7.8	7.8	12.4
			7.0	6.9	11.4
61	5	active	13.6	18.7	17.2
			12.1	17.3	14.8
			10.8	16.1	13.1
			9.7	15.0	11.5
			8.9	14.1	9.6

It was mentioned earlier that it is particularly important when fitting models to data containing missing values to check model assumptions. As with the usual version of multiple regression the most useful diagnostics are the residuals, calculated as the differences between observed values and those predicted by the model. Here each subject, i, will have a vector of residuals, $\mathbf{r}_i$, defined as follows:

$$\mathbf{r}_i = \mathbf{y}_i - \mathbf{X}_i \hat{\boldsymbol{\beta}}, \qquad (6.10)$$

the individual elements of $\mathbf{r}_i$ corresponding to the subject's residual at each time point. One possible method for displaying these residuals is to first calculate each subjects Mahalanobis distances defined thus:

$$D_i^2 = (\mathbf{y}_i - \mathbf{X}_i \hat{\boldsymbol{\beta}})' \hat{\boldsymbol{\Sigma}}^{-1} (\mathbf{y}_i - \mathbf{X}_i \hat{\boldsymbol{\beta}}) \qquad (6.11)$$

If the assumptions of the model, i.e., normality and the form of covariance matrix, are correct these distances have, approximately, a chi-squared distribution with T degrees of freedom (remembering that any missing values will have been imputed before the residuals are calculated). Consequently, a chi-square probability plot of the ordered distances should result in a straight line through the origin. Departures from the assumptions will be indicated by depatures from linearity in this plot.

The chi-squared plots for the Mahalanobis distances from the three models fitted to the data from the oestrogen patch trial are shown in Fig. 6.2. The plot corresponding to the independence model

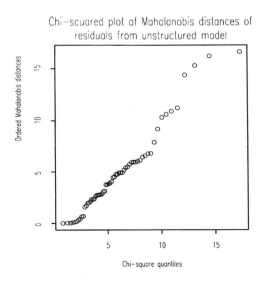

Fig. 6.2(a)

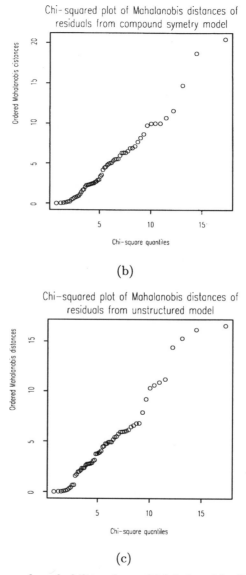

Fig. 6.2. Chi-squared probability plots of Mahalanobis distances from fitting models to the oestrogen patch data. (a) Independence, (b) compound symmetry (c) unstructured.

clearly departs from the expected $y = x$ regression line but both the compound symmetry and unstructured models lead to acceptable plots.

6.5.2. Post-Surgical Recovery in Young Children

In a comparison of the effects of varying doses of an anesthetic on post-surgical recovery, 60 young children undergoing surgery were randomised to receive one of four doses (15, 20, 25 and 30 mg/kg); 15 children were assigned to each dose. Recovery scores were assigned upon admission to the recovery room and at 5, 15 and 30 minutes following admission. The response at each of the four time points was recorded on a six-point scale ranging from 0 (least favourable) to 6 (most favourable). In addition to the doseage, potential covariates were age of patient (in months) and duration of surgery (in minutes). The data are shown in Table 6.6. In this case there are no missing values. Plots of the individual response profiles by treatment group and boxplots of the observations at each time point for each treatment group are shown in Figs. 6.3 and 6.4.

These data will be used to illustrate what is known as a *random coefficients model* in which both the intercept and slope (and possible higher order effects) of each individuals response profile can be modelled as a random effect. Often, data which require a random intercept term can be distinguished from those requiring fixed intercepts by examining plots of the individual response profile (here Fig. 6.3). If individual cases appear as parallel lines, this suggests a random intercept. In a data set requiring a fixed intercept but random slopes, the marginal variance at the end time point will be larger than at earlier time points — the lines spread out with increasing time. A model with both random slope and intercept might begin separated and would spread further, provided the association between slope and intercept was positive. Although Fig. 6.3 is not entirely convincing, here we shall fit a model with both random intercepts and slopes.

Table 6.6. Anaesthesia Recovery Data.

Dose (mg/kg)	Patient	Age (months)	Dur. (min)	Time (min after surgery)			
				0	5	15	30
15	1	36	128	3	5	6	6
15	2	35	70	3	4	6	6
15	3	54	138	1	1	1	4
15	4	47	67	1	3	3	5
15	5	42	55	5	6	6	6
15	6	35	94	3	3	6	6
15	7	30	44	6	6	6	6
15	8	57	54	1	1	1	6
15	9	30	74	1	1	4	6
15	10	41	65	2	2	2	2
15	11	34	50	1	3	3	5
15	12	62	35	3	3	5	6
15	13	24	55	1	1	1	4
15	14	39	165	1	3	5	5
15	15	66	158	0	2	2	3
20	16	22	75	1	1	1	6
20	17	49	42	1	1	1	6
20	18	36	58	2	3	3	6
20	19	43	60	1	1	2	3
20	20	23	64	5	6	6	6
20	21	30	46	1	1	2	4
20	22	9	114	6	6	6	6
20	23	14	50	4	4	6	6
20	24	2	95	1	4	5	5
20	25	50	125	1	2	2	5
20	26	26	127	6	6	6	6
20	27	40	173	0	0	0	4
20	28	12	110	3	6	6	6
20	29	42	47	1	1	5	6
20	30	18	97	2	2	3	5

Table 6.6 (*Continued*)

Dose (mg/kg)	Patient	Age (months)	Dur. (min)	Time (min after surgery)			
				0	5	15	30
25	31	26	103	1	1	0	3
25	32	28	89	3	6	6	6
25	33	41	51	2	3	4	4
25	34	46	93	1	1	5	6
25	35	37	45	2	3	6	6
25	36	28	68	6	6	6	6
25	37	37	35	3	5	6	6
25	38	60	54	2	3	3	6
25	39	60	55	1	1	1	3
25	40	38	78	0	2	6	6
25	41	47	118	0	0	0	0
25	42	38	98	1	1	1	4
25	43	23	58	1	2	6	6
25	44	56	190	1	1	1	1
25	45	31	125	0	3	5	6
30	46	46	72	4	6	6	6
30	47	38	85	2	4	6	6
30	48	59	54	4	5	5	6
30	49	16	100	1	1	1	1
30	50	65	113	2	3	3	5
30	51	53	72	3	4	4	6
30	52	50	70	0	5	5	5
30	53	13	85	0	0	0	4
30	54	17	25	0	0	0	0
30	55	70	53	1	1	1	4
30	56	13	45	0	0	4	6
30	57	60	41	1	1	4	6
30	58	12	61	1	1	4	6
30	59	27	61	3	5	5	6
30	60	56	106	0	1	1	3

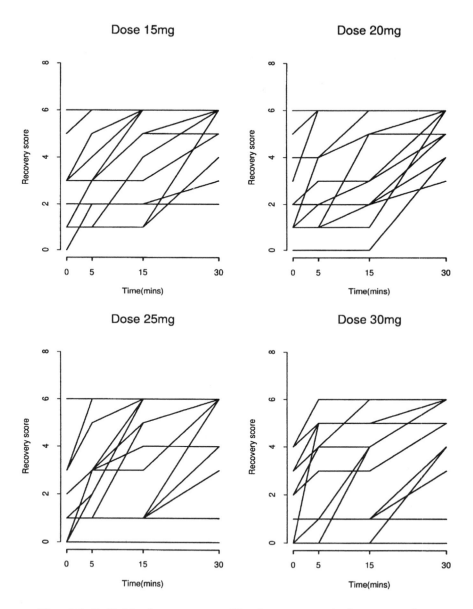

Fig. 6.3. Individual response profiles for post-surgical recovery data.

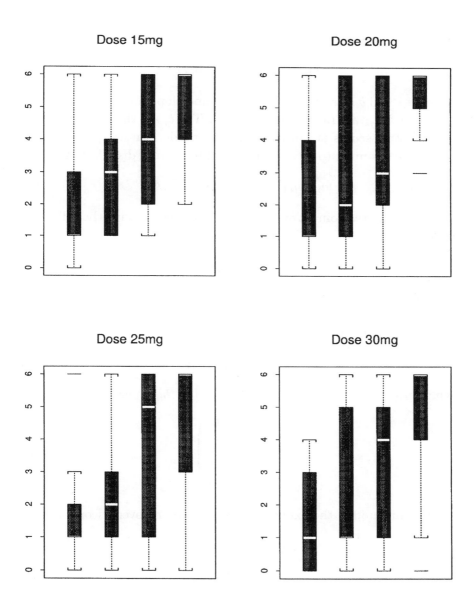

Fig. 6.4. Box-plots of surgical-recovery data.

We assume that the recovery scores for the kth subject at the jth time point and the ith drug dose, y_{ijk}, are given by:

$$y_{ijk} = a_{ik} + b_{ik}t_j + \epsilon_{ijk} \qquad (6.12)$$

where a_{ik} and b_{ik} are random intercept and slope for subject k having dose i, and ϵ_{ijk} are random error terms. The t_j are the times at which the recovery scores are measured. The random intercept and slope terms are assumed to have a multivariate normal distribution:

$$[a_{ik}, b_{ik}]' \sim MVN([\alpha_i, \beta_i]', \boldsymbol{\Phi}) \qquad (6.13)$$

Likewise, the random error terms are assumed to have the following distribution:

$$\epsilon'_{ik} = [\epsilon_{i1k}, \epsilon_{i2k}, \epsilon_{i3k}, \epsilon_{i4k}]' \sim MVN(\mathbf{0}, \sigma^2 \mathbf{I}) \qquad (6.14)$$

The random error terms are assumed to be independent of the random intercepts and slopes.

The model can be written more concisely as:

$$\mathbf{y}_{ik} = \mathbf{Z}\mathbf{u}_{ik} + \epsilon_{ik} \qquad (6.15)$$

where $\mathbf{y}_{ik} = [y_{i1k}, y_{i2k}, y_{i3k}, y_{i4k}]'$, $\mathbf{u}_{ik} = [a_{ik}, b_{ik}]'$ and

$$\mathbf{Z} = \begin{pmatrix} 1 & 0 \\ 1 & 5 \\ 1 & 15 \\ 1 & 30 \end{pmatrix}. \qquad (6.16)$$

Under this model, the expected values of the recovery scores are:

$$E(y_{ijk}) = \alpha_i + \beta_i t_j \qquad (6.17)$$

and the covariance matrix of $\mathbf{y}_{ik}$ has the following *random effects structure*:

$$\boldsymbol{\Sigma} = \mathbf{Z}\boldsymbol{\Phi}\mathbf{Z}' + \sigma^2 \mathbf{I} \qquad (6.18)$$

Table 6.7. Results of Likelihood-based Analysis of Recovery Data (assuming random coefficients model).

Term	df	chi-square	p-value
treatment	3	1.27	0.736
linear time	1	165.88	< 0.001
treatment×time	3	0.10	0.992

The parameter estimates obtained from using BMDP 5V are shown in Table 6.7. To assess differences between the drug groups in intercepts and slopes, *Wald's test* can be used; this assesses whether a particular subset of the parameters, β_m, is zero. The form of this test is:

$$W = \hat{\beta}'_m \mathbf{V}^{-1} \hat{\beta}_m \qquad (6.19)$$

where $\mathbf{V}$ is the covariance matrix of the estimates in the subset of interest. If all m parameters in the subset are zero, then W has a chi-squared distribution with m degrees of freedom.

The results of this test for intercepts and slopes are also shown in Table 6.7. There is no evidence of any difference between the different drug dose groups.

6.6. ANOVA AND MANOVA APPROACHES TO THE ANALYSIS OF LONGITUDINAL DATA

One of the most common types of analysis for longitudinal data, particularly in psychiatry and psychology, remains either univariate or multivariate analysis of variance. The ANOVA approach is usually formulated in terms of a mixed-effects model which includes a random subject effect, this allowing the repeated observations to have the compound symmetry covariance structure. Such a model for the oestrogen patch data takes the form:

$$y_{ijk} = \mu + \alpha_i + \beta_j + \gamma_{ij} + \tau_k + \epsilon_{ijk} \qquad (6.20)$$

where y_{ijk} denotes the depression score of subject k in treatment group i on the jth visit, μ represents an overall mean effect, α_i, $i = 1, 2$ represent the effect of treatment, β_j, $j = 1, \ldots, 6$ represent time effects, and γ_{ij} denotes the group×time interaction. The term τ_k is used for the subject effect specific to subject k, and ϵ_{ijk} represents the usual residual or 'error' terms. The terms α, β and γ are considered fixed effects and both τ and ϵ are assumed to be random effects having normal distributions with zero means and variances θ_1 and θ_2. Such a model implies that the covariance matrix of the repeated observations is as shown in Eq. (6.6).

The MANOVA route removes the constraints on the covariances implied by compound symmetry and allows the covariance matrix of the repeated observations to be fully parameterised as described in the previous section. The problems with assuming compound symmetry and in some situations with allowing an unstructured covariance matrix have been described in Section 6.4. These problems make the use of either ANOVA or MANOVA less than ideal in most situations, although for longitudinal data containing no missing values the latter is unlikely to be seriously misleading. But when the data are affected by dropouts, the application of either ANOVA or MANOVA to complete cases only (still the most usual approach to missing values) should be avoided. If the missing values are MCAR, both approaches do not use the available data as efficiently as they should; much more serious, however, is that if the data are MAR, analysing complete cases only might lead to misleading inferences.

6.7.   INFORMATIVE DROP OUTS

The analyses carried out on the oestrogen patch data in Section 6.4 are only strictly valid if the missing observations caused by the women who dropped out are non-informative. Two questions therefore arise:

- How do we tell whether or not the missing observations are ignorable?
- How do we analyse the data if the missing values are informative?

A number of authors have considered these questions including, Laird (1988), Diggle and Kenward (1994) and Diggle (1998). (Ridout, 1991, considers the slightly simpler problem of testing for completely random dropouts and proposes a method based on logistic regression.) Diggle (1998) proposes an informal approach to assessing whether missing values are likely to be informative or otherwise, involving consideration of the mean profiles of cohorts of completers and those who drop out at particular visits, ignoring the different treatment groups. Figure 6.4 illustrates this proposal on the oestrogen patch example; the completers cohort has steadily decreasing depression scores whereas the cohorts of dropouts have increasing values. (The number of missing values in this example is small so that some of the points plotted in Fig. 6.4 are based on just a few subjects; the plot does however serve to illustrate the general point being made.)

A more formal approach is that suggested by Diggle and Kenward (1994) who propose a modelling framework for longitudinal data with informative dropouts, in which random or completely random dropouts are included as explicit models. A brief technical account of the model is given in Table 6.8, but the essential feature is a logistic model for the probability of dropping out, in which the explanatory variables can include previous values of the response variable as in the model described above, but in addition can include the *unobserved* value at dropout as a latent variable. In other words, the dropout probability is allowed to depend on both the *observed* measurement history and the unobserved value at dropout. The model is implemented in the software OSWALD (see Appendix).

Table 6.8. Diggle and Kenward Model for Dropouts.

- Let $\mathbf{Y}^*$ represent the complete vector of intended measurements and $\mathbf{t} = [t_1, t_2, \ldots, t_n]$ the corresponding set of times at which measurements are taken.
- Let $\mathbf{Y} = [Y_1, Y_2, \ldots, Y_n]$ denote the vector of measurements, with missing values coded as zero.
- $\mathbf{Y}^*$ and $\mathbf{Y}$ coincide as long as the individual remains in the study, implying

$$
\begin{aligned}
Y_k &= Y_k^*, \ k = 1, 2, \ldots, D-1 \\
&= 0 \quad k \geq D
\end{aligned}
$$

where D is a random variable such that $2 \leq D \leq n$ identifies the dropout time and $D = n+1$ identifies no dropout.
- The distribution of $\mathbf{Y}^*$ is assumed to be multivariate normal with probability density function $f^*(\mathbf{y}; \boldsymbol{\beta}, \boldsymbol{\theta})$, where $\boldsymbol{\beta}$ and $\boldsymbol{\theta}$, respectively parameterise the mean and covariance structure of $\mathbf{Y}^*$.
- We assume that the dropout process is such that the probability of dropout at time t_d depends on the history of measurement up to and including t_d.
- For each k, let $\mathbf{H}_k = [y_1, \ldots, y_{k-1}]$ represent the observed history up to time t_{k-1}. The model for the dropout process is then:

$$
\Pr(D = d|\text{history}) = p_d(\mathbf{H}_d, y_d^*; \boldsymbol{\phi})
$$

So the dropout probability depends on both the *observed* measurement history $\mathbf{H}_d$ and the *unobserved* value y_d^*. In addition, the probability depends on a set of parameters $\boldsymbol{\phi}$.
- The equations that determine the joint distribution of $\mathbf{Y}$, and hence the likelihood function of the parameters, $\boldsymbol{\beta}, \boldsymbol{\theta}$ and $\boldsymbol{\phi}$ are:

$$
\Pr(Y_k = 0|\mathbf{H}_k, Y_{k-1} = 0) = 1
$$

$$
\Pr(Y_k = 0|\mathbf{H}_k, Y_{k-1} \neq 0) = \int p_k(\mathbf{H}_k, y; \boldsymbol{\phi}) f_k^*(y|\mathbf{H}_k; \boldsymbol{\beta}, \boldsymbol{\theta}) dy
$$

$$
f_k(y|\mathbf{H}_k; \boldsymbol{\beta}, \boldsymbol{\theta}, \boldsymbol{\phi}) = \{1 - p_k(\mathbf{H}_k, y; \boldsymbol{\phi})\} f_k^*(y|\mathbf{H}_k; \boldsymbol{\beta}, \boldsymbol{\theta}) \ (y \neq 0)
$$

Table 6.8. (*Continued*)

where $f_k^*(y|\mathbf{H}_k; \boldsymbol{\beta}, \boldsymbol{\theta})$ denotes the conditional alternate Gaussian pdf of y_k^* given $\mathbf{H}_k$ and $f_k(y|\mathbf{H}_k; \boldsymbol{\beta}, \boldsymbol{\theta}, \boldsymbol{\phi})$ the conditional pdf of y_k given $\mathbf{H}_k$.

- A linear logistic model is used for $p_k(\mathbf{H}_k, y; \boldsymbol{\phi})$.
- From there the likelihood function for $\boldsymbol{\beta}$, $\boldsymbol{\theta}$ and $\boldsymbol{\phi}$ can be constructed.

(This account is an abbreviated version of that given in Diggle and Kenward, 1994, where readers are referred to for more detail.)

Table 6.9. Results from Diggle–Kenward Model for Dropouts Oestrogen Patch Data (assuming random drop-out based on 1 previous observation).

Analysis method: Maximum likelihood (ML)
Maximised likelihood:
[1] - 1295.658
Mean Parameters:

	(Intercept)	Group	Time	Pre2
PARAMETER	−1.218	−1.751	−0.572	0.807
STD. ERROR	20.58	0.356	0.071	0.094

Dropout parameters:

(Intercept)	$y.d$	$y.d - 1$
−3.941	0	0.103

To illustrate the Diggle–Kenward model for dropouts, the method will be applied to the oestrogen patch example. Part of the outputs from OSWALD corresponding to models for, MAR and informative dropouts are shown in Tables 6.9 and 6.10. The likelihood ratio test for the additional parameter in the informative dropout model indicates that the parameter is not zero. This finding might appear to throw into doubt the previously reported likelihood analyses of these data in which the dropouts were assumed to be non-informative.

Table 6.10. Results from Diggle–Kenward Model for Dropouts Oestrogen Patch Data (assuming informative drop-out).

Maximised likelihood:

[1] - 1291.848

Mean Parameters:

	(Intercept)	Group	Time	Pre2
PARAMETER	10.198	−2.335	−0.670	0.309
STD. ERROR	NA	NA	NA	NA

Dropout parameters:

(Intercept)	$y.d$	$y.d - 1$
−4.797	0.022	0.131

• LR test of additional parameter: 7.62 1d.f.

(The standard errors of the mean parameters for the informative dropout model are not available from OSWALD.)

However, the parameters characterising the mean profiles tell largely the same story in both models. Certainly the likelihood analysis assuming only MAR is less likely to suffer from bias than the alternative of using only complete cases and implicitly assuming MCAR.

The Diggle–Kenward model represents a welcome addition to the methodology available for analysing longitudinal data in which there are dropouts. But as with any new modelling framework, questions need to be asked about its adequacy in practical situations. Matthews (1994), for example, makes the point that if there are many dropouts, the proposed model *can* be applied, but questions whether many statisticians would feel happy to rely on technical virtuosity when 60% of the data are absent. Alternatively, if the proportion of dropouts is low, then much less can be learnt about the dropout process, leading to low power to discriminate between dropout processes. Skinner (1994) suggests that the longitudinal data remaining after dropout may, by themselves, contain very little information about the 'informativeness' of the dropout and concludes that external information about the dropout mechanism be sought and used. A further possible problem identified by Troxel *et al.* (1998) is that bias that results from assuming the wrong type of missingness mechanism may well be more severe than the bias that results from misspecification of a standard full maximum likelihood model.

Despite these and other reservations made in the discussion of Diggle and Kenward's paper, their proposed model does open up the possibility of some almost routine, detailed investigation of the dropout process.

6.8. OTHER METHODS FOR THE ANALYSIS OF LONGITUDINAL DATA

There are a number of methods of analysis that allow for more general covariance matrices to be specified. One, very little used within the clinical trials field, is structural equation modelling (SEM). As typically presented, SEM typically start by a detailed consideration of the appropriate structure for the covariance matrix and only later proceeding to consider the structure of the means that is typically the main focus for the trial analyst. However, a common limitation of SEM software is their limited ability to deal with missing data, typically approached through the fitting of the model to multiple groups, one corresponding to each group of subjects with a common pattern of missing data (see Dunn, Everitt and Pickles, 1993). Rather more practicable are programs such as Mx (Neale, 1995) that perform what is described as full-information maximum-likelihood estimation, that fit the model at the individual subject level if required.

A second increasingly important method uses software for multilevel modelling (e.g., MLWiN — see Appendix). These, too, are capable of fitting models with error covariance matrices with structures like those already described. However, in addition, the appropriate use of dummy variables with random coefficients allows for heteroscedasticity in variances and covariances between treatment groups.

A novel approach to the analysis of longitudinal data is suggested by Tango (1998). Tango postulates that each treatment group consists of a mixture of several distinct latent profiles, a situation he models using a finite mixture model with normal components (see Everitt, 1996). The effect of treatment is characterised by the slope of the latent profiles and the mixing proportions of these latent profiles. An EM algorithm is used for parameter estimation.

Means for dropouts and completers

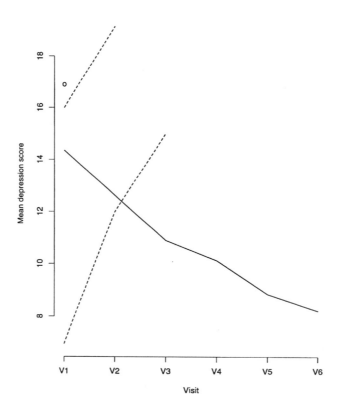

Fig. 6.5. Means for completers and cohorts of subjects dropping out a particular times for oestrogen patch data.

Tango illustrates his proposal on data from a randomised double blind trial of two treatments for chronic hepatitis, a new treatment A, and the standard treatment B. The response variable used was log-transformed serum levels of glutamate pyruvate transaminase (GPT), measured at baseline and at one week intervals up to four weeks. A five-group mixture model was deemed optimal, the groups being labelled, 'greatly improved', 'improved', 'unchanged', 'worsened', 'greatly worsened'. A patient's group membership was determined by the maximum value of their estimated posterior probabilities of belonging to each group. The profiles of all the 124 patients and of the patients in each of the derived groups are shown in Fig. 6.5. The composition of the two-treatment groups in terms of each type of patient was as follows:

Treat- ment	Greatly Improved	Improved	Unchanged	Worsened	Greatly Worsened	Total
A	3	20	17	14	8	62
B	2	13	34	11	2	62

Compared with the standard treatment B, the treatment A has:

- the same proportion of 'greatly improved',
- higher proportion of 'improved',
- higher proportion of 'worsened',
- higher proportion of 'greatly worsened',
- lower proportion of 'unchanged'.

Tango suggests that these characterisations of the efficacy of treatments might be medically important especially for finding the key baseline factors to discriminate responders from non-responders.

6.9. SUMMARY

For longitudinal data where the response variable has a normal distribution, the regression model described in Section 6.4 can be applied

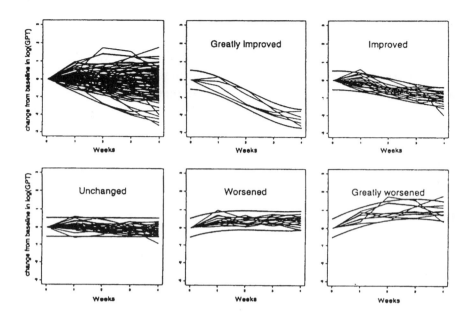

Fig. 6.6. Individual profiles for all patients and for mixture modelling-derived 'types'.

routinely, using software such as PROC MIXED in SAS and BMDP5V. When the data are unbalanced but the missing values can be assumed to be MCAR or MAR, the estimation of the parameters in such models by maximum likelihood provides a completely satisfactory method of analysis and one that is much to be preferred over the commonly used application of univariate or multivariate analysis of variance to complete cases.

Although the missing-at-random assumption made in the likelihood approach described in this chapter is often sensible, Little and Yau (1996) give some examples where it is highly questionable. In such cases, the Diggle–Kenward model for informative dropouts can be applied using the OSWALD package, although at present this should perhaps be regarded as primarily experimental. In addition, Little (1995) suggests that the model may be highly sensitive to model misspecification and in Little and Lau (1996) describes an alternative approach to the dropout problem. Now values of the outcome after dropout are imputed using models for the missing data that condition on all relevant observed data, and in particular on information about treatments actually administered (as opposed to randomised treatment). Following imputation an intention-to-treat analysis based on the treatment as randomised is applied to the imputed data.

Finally, it must be remembered that the proportion of dropouts may, for many trials, be regarded as a measure of the quality of the data produced by the trial. And Lavori's seemingly self-evident statement, "it is always better to have no dropouts" (Lavori, 1992), still has considerable appeal.

CHAPTER 7

Models for Non-Normal Longitudinal Data from Clinical Trials

7.1. INTRODUCTION

In Chapter 4 we gave a brief description of generalised linear models and showed how they have unified regression analysis for discrete and continuous *independent* response variables. An obvious question is how might such models be adapted to be suitable for *correlated* response variables, in particular the repeated measurements taken in a longitudinal study? The multivariate regression model for correlated *normally* distributed response variables found in Chapter 6 provides the first part of the answer, and in this chapter the extension to non-normal responses, in particular, categorical responses, will be considered.

In the linear model for Gaussian data in Chapter 6 *estimation* of the regression parameters needed to take account of the correlations in the data, but their *interpretation* was essentially independent of the correlation structure. One potentially troublesome aspect of modelling non-normal longitudinal data is that this independence of estimation and interpretation no longer always holds. Different assumptions about the source of correlations between the observations can lead to regression coefficients with distinct interpretations as we shall see later. The three principal approaches to introducing correlations are *marginal, random effects* and *transition* models. Each type will now be considered relatively briefly; fuller accounts are available in Diggle, *et al.* (1994).

7.2. MARGINAL MODELS

Longitudinal data can be considered as a series of cross-sections, and marginal models for such data use the generalised linear model discussed in Chapter 4, to fit to each cross-section. In this approach, the relationship of the marginal mean and the explanatory variables is modelled *separately* from the within-subject correlation. Specifically, a marginal model makes the following assumptions:

- $g(\mu_{ij}) = \mathbf{x}'_{ij}\boldsymbol{\beta}$,
- $V_{ij} = \phi V(\mu_{ij})$
- $\text{Corr}(Y_{ij}, Y_{ik}) = \rho(\mu_{ij}, \mu_{ik}; \boldsymbol{\alpha})$, where $\rho(\cdot)$ is a known function and $\boldsymbol{\alpha}$ a set of parameters.

(The nomenclature is that introduced for GLMs in Chapter 4 and for longitudinal data in Chapter 6, with μ_{ij} now representing the expected value of the observation on subject i at time t_j, i.e., Y_{ij}.)

The first two of these assumptions are exactly the same as those made in Chapter 4 for generalised linear models, suitable when only a single response is observed on each subject. The marginal regression coefficients $\boldsymbol{\beta}$ have the same interpretation as coefficients from a cross-sectional analysis, and marginal models are natural analogues for correlated data of generalised linear models for independent data.

Before considering how the parameters in such models can be estimated, it might be helpful to look at a simple example. For this we shall use the respiratory status data introduced in Chapter 5. These data consist of binary observations of whether a patient had good or poor respiratory status at baseline and at each of four post-treatment visits. Two treatment groups were involved and in addition two further covariates, sex and age, were available together with a binary indicator for centre. One possible logistic marginal model is given by:

- $\text{logit}(\mu_{ij}) = \log \frac{\mu_{ij}}{1-\mu_{ij}} = \log \frac{\Pr(Y_{ij}=1)}{\Pr(Y_{ij}=0)} = \beta_0 + \beta_1 \text{treatment}_i,$
- $\text{var}(Y_{ij}) = \mu_{ij}(1 - \mu_{ij}),$
- $\text{Corr}(Y_{ij}, Y_{ik}) = 0$

where treatment_i is a dummy variable indicating the treatment group of subject i.

Here the parameter $\exp(\beta_1)$ is the odds ratio of good respiratory status in the two treatment groups. Since $\exp(\beta_1)$ is a ratio of population frequencies, it is referred to as a *population-averaged* parameter. If all the individuals in the same treatment group have the same probability of good respiratory status, the population frequency is the same as the individual's probability. When, however, there is heterogeneity in the probability in a treatment group, the population frequency is the average of the individual values. (This point will be discussed further later in this chapter.)

By setting the correlation between pairs of observations to zero, we are simply ignoring the likely lack of independence of observations over cross-sections. This is an example of what Davis (1991) refers to as the *independence working model* approach. Although such an approach can yield consistent estimates of the regression parameters in many circumstances, the standard estimators of the variances and covariances of these estimates will not be consistent. This problem can be overcome in a variety of ways, but perhaps the simplest is to make use of an extension of the robust covariance matrix estimator of Huber (1967) and White (1982) (see Chapter 4) that makes it suitable for correlated data.

Fitting the independence working model does not need any specialised software since standard GLM or logistic regression packages can be used. Response measures are organised one per record with each subject contributing as many records as repeated measures.

Table 7.1. Parameter Estimates from an Independence Working Model: Logistic Regression Fitted to the Respiratory Status Data.

Covariate	Estm. Regres. Coefficient	Standard Errors		
		Classical	Robust	Bootstrap
Treatment	1.267	0.235	0.349	0.383
Time	−0.078	0.099	0.082	0.083
Sex	0.137	0.294	0.443	0.482
Age/100	−0.189	0.883	1.305	1.354
Baseline	1.849	0.240	0.349	0.395
Centre	0.651	0.238	0.355	0.372

The bootstrap SE is based on 500 replicates.

The operational simplicity of this approach is hard to exaggerate and Table 7.1 gives the parameter estimates from fitting the following logistic regression model to the respiratory status data given in Table 5.9.

$$\text{logit}(Y_{ij} = 1) = \beta_0 + \beta_1 \text{ treatment}_i + \beta_2 \text{ time}_{ij} + \beta_3 \text{ sex}_i$$

$$+ \beta_4 \text{ age}_i + \beta_5 \text{ centre}_i + \beta_6 \text{ baseline}_i . \qquad (7.1)$$

Three forms of standard error are shown together with their associated test statistic; the classical standard error that is based on the unlikely assumption that the four repeated observations on a subject are independent, the 'robust/sandwich' standard error, and a bootstrap standard error. The bootstrap resampling recognised the repeated measures structure by resampling subjects, each with a set of responses, rather than using single responses. The bootstrap estimate is far closer to the robust/sandwich estimate than the classical estimate, which, for between subjects effects, are much too small. But in the case of the within subjects effects for the time trend over assessment visits, it is the robust and bootstrap estimates that are smaller. Assuming independence is not always anti-conservative.

It is important to keep in mind that what is being estimated by the fitted model is the cross-sectional relationship between variables. Table 7.2 shows the sample frequencies over the joint distribution of the baseline and four trial responses (2 times 16 possible binary response sequences), together with the frequencies predicted by the independence working model given in Eq. (7.1). The other entries in this table will be discussed later. Whilst the time-by-time marginal totals are well fitted by this model, the joint distribution reflected by these response sequences is very poorly fitted. Typical of such data, the sequences with a preponderance of one type of response are more common than expected under the assumption of independence, and the sequences with alternating responses considerably fewer. This should come as no surprise since the model was not fitted to the joint distribution, only to the margins.

Table 7.2. Sample Frequencies and Predicted Frequencies for Respiratory Status Data.

Response	Observed Frequency	Independence Working Model	Transition Model	Random Effects Model
Baseline 0				
0000	25	13.3	14.3	21.9
0001	2	4.3	4.1	3.1
0010	4	4.6	4.6	3.5
0011	0	2.3	3.0	1.4
0100	2	5.0	5.6	4.0
0101	0	2.5	2.9	1.6
0110	2	2.7	3.7	1.8
0111	4	2.1	4.1	1.7
1000	3	5.4	4.2	4.5
1001	0	2.7	1.7	1.8
1010	1	2.9	2.0	2.0
1011	2	2.2	1.8	1.9
1100	2	3.2	2.2	2.2

Table 7.2. (*Continued*)

Response	Observed Frequency	Independence Working Model	Transition Model	Random Effects Model
1101	3	2.4	1.6	2.2
1110	1	2.6	2.1	2.5
1111	10	2.7	3.2	5.0
Baseline 1				
0000	1	0.3	0.2	0.4
0001	0	0.5	0.3	0.4
0010	0	0.6	0.3	0.5
0011	3	1.2	0.6	0.7
0100	1	0.6	0.6	0.6
0101	0	1.3	0.9	0.8
0110	1	1.4	0.9	0.9
0111	1	4.0	2.4	2.6
1000	4	0.7	1.1	0.6
1001	2	1.4	1.8	0.9
1010	1	1.5	1.6	1.0
1011	3	4.3	3.9	3.0
1100	0	1.6	3.1	1.2
1101	1	4.6	5.7	3.4
1110	5	5.0	5.5	3.8
1111	27	21.0	21.2	29.2

7.2.1. Marginal Modelling using Generalised Estimating Equations

The independence working model used above can be estimated using the approach outlined for generalised linear models in Chapter 4. But for more complex marginal models in which we wish to take advantage of the correlation between pairs of observations to obtain more efficient estimates of the regression parameters, we need to consider a new procedure introduced by Liang and Zeger (1986), and known as *generalised estimating equations* (GEE). This approach may be

viewed as a multivariate extension of the generalised linear model
and the quasi-likelihood method (see Chapter 4). The use of the
latter leads to consistent inferences about mean responses without
requiring specific assumptions to be made about second and higher
order moments. In this way intractable likelihood functions with possibly many nuisance parameters, in addition to β and α, are avoided.
A brief account of GEE is given in Table 7.3. More detailed accounts
are available in Liang and Zeger (1986) and Zeger, Liang and Prentice (1988). (Software for fitting GEE models is discussed in the
Appendix.)

Table 7.3. Generalised Estimating Equations.

- In the absence of a likelihood function, Liang and Zeger (1986) show
  that the parameters of a generalised linear model for longitudinal data,
  β and α, can be otained from a multivariate analogue of the quasilikelihood mentioned briefly in Chapter 4.
- The generalised estimating equation is given by:

$$\mathbf{U}(\beta, \alpha) = \sum_{i=1}^{n} \left(\frac{\partial \mu_i(\beta)}{\partial \beta} \right)' \mathbf{V}_i^{-1} (\mathbf{y}_i - \mu_i(\beta)) = \mathbf{0}$$

- $\mathbf{V}_i$ is assumed to be of the form:

$$\mathbf{V}_i = \mathbf{\Delta}_i^{1/2} \mathbf{R}_i(\alpha) \mathbf{\Delta}_i^{1/2} / \phi$$

  where $\mathbf{\Delta}_i$ is a diagonal matrix of variances, the elements of which depend on the elements of μ_i, and $\mathbf{R}_i(\alpha)$ is a working correlation matrix.
- Some possibilities for $\mathbf{R}_i(\alpha)$ are:

  (a) An identity matrix leading to the independence working model in
      which the generalised estimating equation reduces to the univariate
      estimating equation given in Chapter 4, obtained by assuming that
      the elements of $\mathbf{y}_i$ are independent.

  (b) An *exchangeable* correlation matrix with a single parameter similar
      to that described in Chapter 6. Here corr$(Y_{ij}, Y_{ik}) = \alpha$.

  (c) An AR–1 *autoregressive* correlation matrix, also with a single pa-
      rameter, but in which corr$(Y_{ij}, Y_{ik}) = \alpha^{|k-j|}$, $j \neq k$.

Table 7. (*Continued*)

(d) An unstructured correlation matrix with $T(T-1)/2$ parameters in which $\text{corr}(Y_{ij}, Y_{ik}) = \alpha_{jk}$.

- In cases of possible overdispersion, the scale parameter ϕ can again be estimated by the moments estimator mentioned in Chapter 4, using observation specific Pearson residuals, $\hat{r}_{ij}$.

- One version of GEE also uses moment estimators for the correlation parameters. For the exchangeable model, for example,

$$\hat{\alpha} = \hat{\phi}\frac{\sum_i\sum_{k>j}\hat{r}_{ij}\hat{r}_{ik}}{\{\sum_i[n_i(n_i-1)/2]-p\}}$$

- The estimation process then consists of an iteration between iterative weighted least squares estimation of the regression parameters for a given estimate of the correlation parameters, followed by a recalculation of the latter based on the residuals from the current estimates of the former.

- Other approaches to GEE estimation are described in Zhao and Prentice (1990) and Prentice and Zhao (1991).

- The GEE method produces consistent estimators for β and its covariance matrix without requiring: (a) specification of the joint distribution of the repeated observations for each individual; (b) correct specification of the correlation structure in $\mathbf{U}(\beta, \alpha)$.

Table 7.4 presents results from logistic regression models fitted to the respiratory status data using GEE under a variety of assumptions about the correlational structure. It is sufficient for our purposes to present results only for the treatment effect of main interest, and the trend over occasions — the only variable that varies within subjects. Both classical and robust standard errors are given, although we should now expect the differences between these two standard error estimators to be smaller since, unlike the independence working model used earlier, these models all make at least a plausible assumption as to the correlation structure (marked differences might have suggested possible model misspecification).

Table 7.4. Results from Fitting Logistic Regression Model to Respiratory Status Data under Various Assumptions about Correlational Structure.

Covariate	Model	Estimate	Classical SE	z-test	Robust SE	z-test
Treatment	Exch	1.256	0.331	3.79	0.348	3.61
	AR–1	1.205	0.308	3.91	0.349	3.45
	Unstr	1.239	0.330	3.76	0.347	3.58
Time	Exch	−0.078	0.081	−0.97	0.082	−0.95
	AR–1	−0.097	0.101	−0.96	0.083	−1.18
	Unstr	−0.086	0.085	−1.01	0.082	−1.05

Table 7.5 gives the lower triangle of the estimated correlation matrices from each of these models. The estimated correlations from the unstructured model look to be closer to those of an exchangeable structure than the autoregressive (AR–1) structure. In the latter model, the correlation between pairs of observations are expected to decline with separation in time much more quickly than they actually appear to do, whereas the exchangeable model assumes that this correlation remains constant. This greater similarity, in this case, of the unstructured and exchangeable models as compared to the AR–1 model, is also reflected in the estimated regression coefficients and standard errors.

Nonetheless all the models give similar findings, with there being little doubt as to the presence of a treatment effect and there being little trend over assesment visit.

Table 7.6 presents some well known data originally presented by Thall and Vail (1990) involving a clinical trial of treatment for epilepsy in which a total of 59 patients were randomly allocated to either a placebo or the active treatment, namely the drug progabide. In this trial, the response variable was a count of the number of seizures within four successive intervals of two weeks. A baseline

Table 7.5. Estimated Correlation Matrices for the Respiratory Status Data.

(a) *Exchangeable*

$$\hat{\mathbf{R}} = \begin{pmatrix} 1.00 & & & \\ 0.33(0.18) & 1.00 & & \\ 0.33(0.18) & 0.33(0.18) & 1.00 & \\ 0.33(0.18) & 0.33(0.18) & 0.33(0.18) & 1.00 \end{pmatrix}$$

(b) *AR–1*

$$\hat{\mathbf{R}} = \begin{pmatrix} 1.00 & & & \\ 0.38 & 1.00 & & \\ 0.15 & 0.38 & 1.00 & \\ 0.06 & 0.15 & 0.38 & 1.00 \end{pmatrix}$$

(c) *Unstructured*

$$\hat{\mathbf{R}} = \begin{pmatrix} 1.00 & & & \\ 0.32 & 1.00 & & \\ 0.20 & 0.42 & 1.00 & \\ 0.29 & 0.34 & 0.38 & 1.00 \end{pmatrix}$$

measure of the response was also taken and, in addition, the age of each patient was recorded. Figure 7.1 is a plot of the log of the total number of seizures (plus one) during the trial against the log of the baseline seizure count. Except for subject 58, with an unusually low number of seizures during the trial, the relationship looks plausibly linear on this log scale. The plot also suggests that subject 49 is likely to have high influence.

The difference in mean log-total for placebo and treatment groups (3.21 — s.e. 0.16 and 2.80 — s.e. 0.19) of 0.41 was not significantly different from zero using a simple *t*-test. Of course, controlling for baseline differences improves efficiency. However, A

Table 7.6. Data from a Clinical Trial of Patients Suffering from Epilepsy.

ID	y_1	y_2	y_3	y_4	Treatment	Baseline	Age
1	5	3	3	3	0	11	31
2	3	5	3	3	0	11	30
3	2	4	0	5	0	6	25
4	4	4	1	4	0	8	36
5	7	18	9	21	0	66	22
6	5	2	8	7	0	27	29
7	6	4	0	2	0	12	31
8	40	20	23	12	0	52	42
9	5	6	6	5	0	23	37
10	14	13	6	0	0	10	28
11	26	12	6	22	0	52	36
12	12	6	8	4	0	33	24
13	4	4	6	2	0	18	23
14	7	9	12	14	0	42	36
15	16	24	10	9	0	87	26
16	11	0	0	5	0	50	26
17	0	0	3	3	0	18	28
18	37	29	28	29	0	111	31
19	3	5	2	5	0	18	32
20	3	0	6	7	0	20	21
21	3	4	3	4	0	12	29
22	3	4	3	4	0	9	21
23	2	3	3	5	0	17	32
24	8	12	2	8	0	28	25
25	18	24	76	25	0	55	30
26	2	1	2	1	0	9	40
27	3	1	4	2	0	10	19
28	13	15	13	12	0	47	22
29	11	14	9	8	1	76	18
30	8	7	9	4	1	38	32

Table 7.6. Data from a Clinical Trial of Patients Suffering from Epilepsy.

ID	y_1	y_2	y_3	y_4	Treatment	Baseline	Age
31	0	4	3	0	1	19	20
32	3	6	1	3	1	10	30
33	2	6	7	4	1	19	18
34	4	3	1	3	1	24	24
35	22	17	19	16	1	31	30
36	5	4	7	4	1	14	35
37	2	4	0	4	1	11	27
38	3	7	7	7	1	67	20
39	4	18	2	5	1	41	22
40	2	1	1	0	1	7	28
41	0	2	4	0	1	22	23
42	5	4	0	3	1	13	40
43	11	14	25	15	1	46	33
44	10	5	3	8	1	36	21
45	19	7	6	7	1	38	35
46	1	1	2	3	1	7	25
47	6	10	8	8	1	36	26
48	2	1	0	0	1	11	25
49	102	65	72	63	1	151	22
50	4	3	2	4	1	22	32
51	8	6	5	7	1	41	25
52	1	3	1	5	1	32	35
53	18	11	28	13	1	56	21
54	6	3	4	0	1	24	41
55	3	5	4	3	1	16	32
56	1	23	19	8	1	22	26
57	2	3	0	1	1	25	21
58	0	0	0	0	1	13	36
59	1	4	3	2	1	12	37

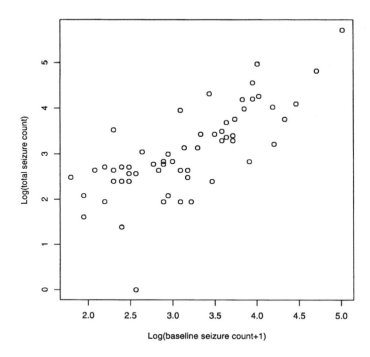

Fig. 7.1. Plot of log of total number of seizures (plus one) against log of the baseline seizure count for epilepsy data in Table 7.6.

Cook–Heisberg test identified heteroscedasticity in a regression of log-total on treatment group, log-baseline and age, suggesting the need to use the Huberized/robust/sandwich (heteroscedasticity consistent) parameter covariance estimator in making inference about effects in such a model. This suggested a significant treatment effect conditional upon covariates of -0.38 with a 95% confidence interval of $(-0.71, -0.05)$.

We have already noted in Chapter 4 how regression analyses of log transformed data can be distorted by obervations with responses at or close to 0. Subject 58 is clearly one such case. Perhaps the natural model to analyse count data such as these is some form of GLM based on a Poisson error distribution. However, fitting a GLM with covariates for treatment, age and log-baseline,

Table 7.7. GEE Poisson Regression Estimates for the Epilepsy Data.

Covariate	Model	Estimate	SE	z-test
Treatment	(1) Indep with robust	−0.031	0.193	−0.163
	(2) Exch	−0.025	0.071	−0.361
	(3) Exch with overdisp	−0.025	0.155	−0.164
	(4) Exch with overdisp and robust	−0.025	0.193	−0.133
	(5) AR–1 with overdisp	−0.035	0.149	−0.233
	(6) Unstructured with overdisp	−0.035	0.154	−0.226
Time	(1) Indep with robust	−0.059	0.016	−3.76
	(2) Exch	−0.059	0.016	−3.743
	(3) Exch with overdisp	−0.059	0.035	−1.704
	(4) Exch with overdisp and robust	−0.059	0.035	−1.670
	(5) AR–1 with overdisp	−0.064	0.044	−1.438
	(6) Unstructured with overdisp	−0.056	0.039	−1.226

with a log link function and Poisson errors to the total seizure count gave a Pearson model chi-square of 614.79 for 55 degrees of freedom, clearly indicating some form of overdispersion. As we shall see, this has implications for the specification of any GEE model that we might fit as part of a longitudinal analysis of the four separate trial counts.

Table 7.7 shows the results for treatment effect and for the trend over visit from models with a log link, Poisson errors and additional covariates for log-baseline and age which, for the sake of clarity, have not been reported in the table. For illustrative purposes, the fitted model included simple main effects and a common pattern of overdispersion, though Thall and Vail (1990) find some evidence in favour of a more complicated structure. We show results from six models:

(1) an independence working model with robust standard errors,
(2) an exchangeable correlation model,
(3) as in (2) but with the scale parameter estimated by the Pearson chi-square/residual divided by the degrees of freedom in order to allow for overdispersion,
(4) an exchangeable model with robust standard errors,
(5) a first-order autoregressive model allowing for overdispersion,
(6) a model with an unstructured correlation matrix allowing for overdispersion.

Unlike the previous example, the results from the basic exchangeable model (2) are quite different from those of the independence working model with robust standard errors (1). However, this is not because the exchangeable correlation matrix is grossly innappropriate (though it is not especially good). Rather, as the results from model (3) show, it is because model (2) has not allowed for overdispersion. It is clear that at least as much thought must be given to the possible presence of overdispersion as to the structure of the correlation matrix. The use of the robust standard errors will cope with failures in either, and as we see from model (4), their use with the overdispersed exchangeable model does increase the standard error for the treatment effect beyond the value of the classical standard error from the overdispersed model. The AR–1 Model (5) and the unstructured or free correlation Model (6) give quite similar results. Inspection of the table of estimated correlations from Model (6), explains why. Unlike in the respiratory disease example, the estimated pattern is suggestive of an autoregressive rather than an exchangeable correlation matrix.

The results from all these GEE models differ strikingly from the results based on applying regression to the log-transformed counts. This very much reflects the variation in the relative influence that is attached to a small number of datapoints according to the particular mean-variance relationship assumed, a circumstance previously illustrated using the polyp count data in Chapter 4. The analyses

Table 7.8. Estimated Correlation Matrix for Epilepsy Data.

Unstructured

$$\hat{\mathbf{R}} = \begin{pmatrix} 1.00 & & & \\ 0.44 & 1.00 & & \\ 0.39 & 0.57 & 1.00 & \\ 0.24 & 0.30 & 0.41 & 1.00 \end{pmatrix}$$

illustrate that in general, for trials with a comparable subjects by time structure, a greater emphasis should probably be placed in the use of model comparisons and diagnostics to examine the issues relating to dispersion in longitudinal GLMs than to those relating to the details of the correlation structure.

7.3. RANDOM EFFECTS MODELS

The essential feature of a random effects model for longitudinal data is that there is natural heterogeneity across individuals in their regression coefficients and that this heterogeneity can be represented by an appropriate probability distribution. Correlation among observations from one person arises from them sharing unobservable variables. In the respiratory status data, for example, variation in the propensity to have poor respiratory status might, in this instance, merely reflect variation in severity of illness not captured by the simple binary response. For a random effects model, the assumptions of the marginal generalised linear model are modified to:

- $g(\mu_{ij}^c) = \mathbf{x}_{ij}'\boldsymbol{\beta}^* + \mathbf{d}_{ij}'\boldsymbol{\tau}_i,$
- $V_{ij}^C = \phi v(\mu_{ij}^c)$

where μ_{ij}^c is the expected value of Y_{ij} conditional on the values of unobserved (latent) random variables τ_i, specific to subject i; V_{ij}^c is the corresponding conditional variance. The term $\mathbf{d}_{ij}$ is a vector of explanatory variables; for example, if $\mathbf{d}'_{ij} = [1, t_{ij}]$, then the elements of τ_i correspond to the intercept and slope of a subject specific time-trend in the mean response. We use β^* here rather than β, to emphasise that the substantive meaning of the regression parameter is different from that of β in a marginal model, unless the response variable has a normal distribution. To illustrate this difference, we will use the following simple random effects logistic regression model:

$$\text{logit}(Y_{ij} = 1|\tau_i) = \beta_0^* + \beta_1^* x_{ij} + \tau_i \tag{7.2}$$

where $\tau_i \sim N(0, \sigma^2)$. It is convenient for our purposes here to rewrite this as:

$$\text{logit}(Y_{ij} = 1|U_i) = \beta_0^* + \beta_1^* x_{ij} + \sigma U_i \tag{7.3}$$

where $U_i \sim N(0, 1)$. The parameter σ is a measure of the degree of heterogeneity between subjects because the *subject-specific* intercepts are $\beta_0^* + \sigma U_i$, $i = 1, \ldots, n$, and the U_i have a standard normal distribution. In this model, the regression parameter β_1^* must be interpreted *conditionally* on the subject's own value of U_i. Zeger, Diggle and Huang (1998) derive the marginal properties of the random effects model in Eq. (7.3), so that the population-averaged coefficient of the former can be compared with the subject-specific effect of the latter. This requires integrating out the dependence on the unobserved U_i; so, for example, the unconditional mean response is:

$$\Pr(Y_{ij} = 1) = \int \Pr(Y_{ij} = 1|u) f(u) du \tag{7.4}$$

$$= \int \frac{\exp(\beta_0^* + \beta_1^* x_{ij} + \sigma u)}{1 + \exp(\beta_0^* + \beta_1^* x_{ij} + \sigma u)} f(u) du \tag{7.5}$$

where $f(\cdot)$ is the standard normal density function. Using an approximation for the integral, Zeger *et al.* (1988) show that:

$$\text{logit}(Y_{ij} = 1) \approx (c^2 \sigma^2 + 1)^{-1/2} (\beta_0^* + \beta_1^* x_{ij}) \tag{7.6}$$

where $c = 16\sqrt{3}/(15\pi)$; consequently,

$$\beta \approx (c^2 \sigma^2 + 1)^{-1/2} \beta^* \tag{7.7}$$

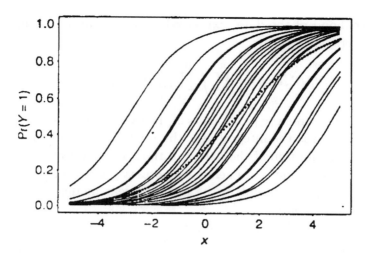

Fig. 7.2. Simulation of the probability of a positive response in a random intercept model logit $\Pr(Y_{ij} = 1|U_i) = -1.0 + x_{ij} + 1.5U_i$ where U_i is a standard normal variable. The dotted line is the average over all 25 subjects (taken with permission from Zeger, Diggle and Huang, 1998).

where $c^2 \approx 0.346$. Zeger, Diggle and Huang (1998) demonstrate this 'shrinkage' effect by simulation. Figure 7.2 shows their results obtained by assuming $\beta_0^* = -1$, $\beta_1^* = 1$ and $\sigma = 1.5$. The dashed lines show $\Pr(Y_{ij} = 1|U_i)$ as functions of x for each of 25 subjects, whilst the solid line shows $\Pr(Y_{ij} = 1)$, calculated as the average of all 25 subject-specific functions. The solid line, which is in effect what we would be estimating in a marginal model, is very well approximated by a linear logistic, but with regression parameter β_1 substantially smaller that β_1^*, as predicted by Eq. (7.7).

In practice, there is general agreement that average effects are often of interest from a public health point of view, but may not be so pertinent where the interest lies in scientific investigation of the individual level process or in individual level prediction.

For a random effects extension of the GLM, it is possible to estimate parameters using traditional maximum likelihood methods.

The likelihood of the data, expressed as a function of the unknown parameters, is given by:

$$L(\boldsymbol{\beta}^*, \boldsymbol{\alpha}; \mathbf{y}) = \prod_{i=1}^{n} \int \prod_{i=1}^{n_i} f_{ij}(y_{ij}|\tau) f(\tau; \boldsymbol{\alpha}) d\tau \qquad (7.8)$$

where $\boldsymbol{\alpha}$ represents the parameters of the random effects distribution. The likelihood is the integral over the unobserved random effects of the joint distribution of the data and the random effects. Numerical integration techniques are generally necessary to evaluate the likelihood in Eq. (7.8), except in the case of linear models for normally distributed responses.

As an illustration of the use of a random effects model, the following logistic regression model will be fitted to the respiratory status data:

$$\text{logit}(Y_{ij} = 1|\tau) = \beta_0 + \beta_1 \text{ treatment}_i + \beta_2 \text{ time}_{ij} + \beta_3 \text{ sex}_i$$

$$+ \beta_4 \text{ age}_i + \beta_5 \text{ centre}_i + \beta_6 \text{ baseline}_i + \tau_i . \quad (7.9)$$

For this model, a likelihood conditional upon τ for a subject is of the form:

$$L(\mathbf{y}_i|\boldsymbol{\beta}x, \tau) = \prod_{j=1}^{4} [\Pr(y_{ij} = 1|\boldsymbol{\beta}x, \tau)^{y_{ij}} \Pr(y_{ij} = 0|\tau)^{1-y_{ij}}]. \quad (7.10)$$

This likelihood can be averaged over some distribution for τ and then maximised over subjects to obtain the required regression coefficient estimates. A variety of distributional forms for τ might be assumed. Table 7.9 shows the results in which the random effect τ has been assumed to be normally distributed. The integral calculation was approximated by the use of 8-point Gaussian quadrature.

The significance of the effects as estimated by this random effects model and by the GEE models of Tables 7.7 is generally similar. However, as expected from the discussion above, the estimated coefficients are substantially larger. Thus, while the estimated effect of treatment of a randomly sampled individual, given the set

Table 7.9. Results from Random Effects Logistic Regression Model Fitted to Respiratory Status Data.

Covariate	Estimate	SE	z	p-value
Treatment	2.14	0.572	3.74	$< .001$
Visit	-0.12	0.125	-0.99	0.3
Sex	0.32	0.662	0.48	0.6
Age/100	-2.45	2.001	-1.23	0.2
Baseline	2.90	0.616	4.71	< 0.001
Centre	0.84	0.573	1.46	0.1

of observed covariates, was estimated by the marginal models to increase the log-odds of being disease free by 1.3, the estimate from the random effects model is 2.3. These are not inconsistent results but reflect the fact that the models are estimating different parameters. The random effects estimator is conditional upon each patient's random effect, a quantity that is rarely known in practice. Were we to examine the log-odds of the average predicted probabilities with and without treatment (averaged over the random effect), this would give an estimate comparable to that estimated within the marginal model.

In terms of covariate effects, the parameterisation of this random effects model corresponds to the marginal model considered in Section 7.2. The model is, however, now a model of the *joint* responses, and as the tabulated predicted frequencies in Table 7.2 show, the introduction of the random effect has captured the pattern of persistence in response remarkably well.

7.4. TRANSITION MODELS

In a transition GLM, correlation amongst the observations is assumed to arise from the dependence of the present observation on one or more past values. Here we model the mean and variance of

Y_{ij} conditional on past responses Y_{ij-k}, for $k \geq 1$. The assumptions of a cross-sectional GLM would now be replaced by:

- $g(\mu_{ij}^t) = \mathbf{x}_{ij}\boldsymbol{\beta} + \sum_{k=1}^r \alpha_k y_{ij-k}$,
- $V_{ij}^t = \phi v(\mu_{ij}^t)$

where now μ_{ij}^t and V_{ij}^t are the expectation and variance of Y_{ij} conditional on all Y_{ij-k} for $k \geq 1$:

An example of a simple transition model for the respiratory status data is:

$$\text{logit}(Y_{ij} = 1) = \beta_0 + \beta_1 \text{ treatment}_i + \alpha Y_{ij-1} \quad j = 1, \ldots, 4 \quad (7.11)$$

Here the chance of respiratory status being good at a particular time point depends on the treatment group and also on whether or not a subject's respiratory status was good or not at the previous visit. The parameter $\exp(\alpha)$ is the odds ratio of good respiratory status amongst subjects having good and poor status at the previous visit. The parameter $\exp(\beta_1)$ is now interpreted as the odds ratio for good respiratory status in the two treatment groups, for patients with the same prior (or lag minus one) respiratory status. This odds ratio can therefore be considered as applying to the transition rates among states of respiratory disorder.

Table 7.10 presents a cross-tabulation by treatment group of the respiratory status at time t, given the immediately prior status. In the placebo group, the simple transition rates from poor to good and from good to poor are roughly comparable, being 0.21, and 0.27 respectively. In the active treatment group, however, these two transition rates are more divergent, that from poor to good being 0.37 and that from good to poor 0.15. Thus, while the pattern is consistent with the hypothesis that the active treatment might benefit those with respiratory problems, it also suggests that the treatment may be of no benefit to those without problems — the treatment may not be preventative.

Table 7.10. Cross-Tabulation of Response Patterns for Respiratory Disorder Data.

Placebo

	$Y_{t-1} = 0$	$Y_{t-1} = 1$	Total
$Y_t = 0$	100	27	127
Column %	79.4	26.5	
$Y_t = 1$	26	75	101
Column %	20.6	73.5	
Total	126	102	228

Active

	$Y_{t-1} = 0$	$Y_{t-1} = 1$	Total
$Y_t = 0$	49	20	69
Column %	62.8	14.5	
$Y_t = 1$	29	118	147
Column %	37.2	85.5	
Total	78	138	216

To investigate this possibility in more detail, we fitted a logistic regression model which included the lagged response as an explanatory variable, e.g.,

$$\text{logit}(Y_{ij}) = \beta_0 + \beta_1 \text{ treatment}_i + \beta_2 Y_{ij-1} + \beta_3 \text{ treatment}_i \times Y_{ij-1}$$

$$(7.12)$$

Transition models can be fitted by maximising the conditional likelihood of $Y_{i2}, \ldots, Y_{it_i}$ given Y_{i1}. Such models can be fitted using standard GLM software. The estimated ordinary and Huberised standard errors are shown in Table 7.11. The latter are 10–20% larger than the former; this suggests that the correlation in these observations has not been fully accounted for by the inclusion of the immediately prior response and that second and higher order terms might be required. However, the treatment by prior status interaction term is

Table 7.11. Results from Fitting Transition Model Logistic Regression to Respiratory Status Data.

Covariate	Estimate	Classical SE	Robust SE
Treatment	0.822	0.321	0.380
Y_{t-1}	2.369	0.314	0.384
Interaction	−0.010	0.461	0.568

Table 7.12. Results from Exchangeable Marginal Logistic Regression Status with Effects of Lagged (Prior) Respiratory Status.

Covariate	Estimate	Classical SE	z-test
Treatment	1.003	0.287	3.49
Visit	−0.186	0.091	−2.04
baseline status	0.973	0.301	3.24
lagged status	1.831	0.279	6.57

neither large nor at all significant, whereas the main effect of the treatment (and prior history) is both.

The use of robust standard errors in the previous table could be thought of as applying an IWM marginal modelling strategy to a transition model. Equally, we could have approached the analysis by adding the lagged response to the covariate list of a previous marginal model. We did just that to the model of Eq. (7.1), and Table 7.12 gives the estimates for a subset of the estimated effects. Comparison with Table 7.4 shows the estimated effect of treatment to be slightly reduced, and the lagged respiratory status as a significant predictor, its effect being in addition to that for the baseline response.

We have tabulated the expected frequencies for this model in Table 7.2 for comparison with the corresponding simple marginal model without lagged effects and the random effects model. In this instance, as a method of modelling the joint response distribution, there is little that has been gained by the addition of the lagged response, particularly in comparison with the random effects model. This is perhaps not surprising given the evidence from previous analyses that an exchangeable model fits the data better than an autoregressive one, and that the chosen random effects model corresponds to an assumption of an exchangeable correlation, while the transition model corresponds rather more to the autoregressive pattern.

7.5.   A COMPARISON OF METHODS

The way in which we have tackled the preceeding example indicates that a mixing of the various approaches to the analysis of non-normal longitudinal data is perfectly possible. It is, however, something that we would suggest be used in practice only with some caution. This stems largely from the rather different philopsophical bases of the different modelling approaches, since as outlined in Section 7.3, the different approaches do not attempt to estimate the same effect. Marginal models only rarely correspond to a probability model for the process, but nonetheless are straightforward to apply and do estimate the effects that are seemingly of immediate interest. However, they should not be chosen uncritically, and a number of authors have questioned the value of the parameter estimates from such models (e.g., Lindsey and Lampert, 1997), particularly where lagged response variables are included.

Transition and random effects models are typically put forward as probability models. When specified correctly, their structure is one such that they could be used to simulate data with the same properties as those of the data under study, and the parameters that are estimated potentially (but not always nor necessarily) have a causal interpretation. To specify such models correctly, the investigator can and should draw upon available clinical and scientific knowledge of the disease. However, the difficulties in achieving correct model specifications are considerable, particularly where it is wished that a full causal interpretation be placed on all the parameter estimates. To illustrate this point, consider a typical random effects model in which the lagged response is used as a covariate. The random effect in a typical random intercept model is included to account for between-subjects variations in response propensity, and as such is clearly correlated with response, both current and past. Thus, although the routine method for estimating random effects models assumes that the random effect is uncorrelated with all included regressors, in general, this is unlikely to be the case where the covariate list includes lagged responses. This sort of issue has been explored rather more in social and economic applications of random effects models than in clinical trial settings (e.g., Chesher and Lancaster, 1983; Pickles, 1991).

Even when properly specified, it may be the case that a population average estimate of treatment effect, rather than a fully conditional estimate, may be required to assist in assessing results for their implications for public health. However, such population average estimates are easy to obtain by averaging the estimated impact of treatment (on whatever scale is desired) for each subject over the study sample. Of course, this assumes that the study sample is representative of the target population, but this is anyway implicit in the interpretation given to the parameters of marginal models as being population average estimates.

Overall therefore, although there is currently a strong preference for the use of marginal models, the case for them is not so overwhelming that they should be used to the exclusion of others. Indeed, in some respects the debate as to the use of these different methods for longitudinal analysis within clinical trials has hardly begun.

7.6.   MISSING DATA AND WEIGHTED ESTIMATING EQUATIONS

The generalised estimating-equation approach described in Section 7.2.1 is not a full likelihood method but it is valid when data are missing completely at random. The issue of bias of the GEE, when the data are not MCAR, has been discussed by Kenward *et al.* (1994). Robins and Rotnitzky (1995) have modified the GEE method, allowing it to be valid under the weaker assumption that the data are missing at random. The modification in part involves weighting the usual GEE by the inverse of the estimated probabilities of 'missingness' for each subject. These probabilities can be derived from a logistic (or probit) model of response in which observed outcomes and/or other observed measures are covariates.

7.6.1. Missing Data in a Longitudinal Clinical Trial with an Ordinal Response

Table 7.13 presents longitudinal data from a clinical trial in which the response was measured on an ordinal scale of severity (0 = good, 3 = poor) in relation to recovery from sprain injury. The principal interest here lies in the impact of treatment on speeding-up the process of recovery, i.e., a time by treatment interaction.

One relatively straightforward method of analysis is to use a proportional odds model (see Chapter 4) and to tackle the repeated measures aspect of the problem using the marginal modelling approach, most simply by assuming an independence working model (or the essentially equivalent methods of survey research). The only terms in the model that we will examine are those for treatment, a linear trend for occasion and their interaction. Any correlation over time is not being formally modelled.

However, before considering the results, an inspection of Table 7.12 indicates that by the end of the trial, 9 out of the 30 participants had dropped out. We compare three approaches to tackling this problem of missing data. The first method uses all the available observations and requires that we assume that the missing observations are missing completely at random. The second method uses 'last observation carried forward' to 'fill-in' missing observations.

Table 7.13. Recovery from Sprain Injury.

Treatment Group		Control group	
Patient ID	Pain scores	Patient ID	Pain scores
1	211*	17	3000
2	21*0	18	11*0
3	1100	19	2220
4	110*	20	1100
5	2100	21	2210
6	21**	22	110*
7	210*	23	2222
8	2100	24	210*
9	200*	25	2100
10	2110	26	3221
11	3221	27	22*0
12	3221	28	222*
13	3210	29	2211
14	3233	30	2211
15	332*		
16	3211		

* = missing value.

The third method adopts an inverse probability weighting approach in which adjustments are made for selective loss of patients as reflected in differences in any measures made prior to loss. In this method, the complete observations at times 1 and 2 receive a weight of 1. For occasion 3, weights were obtained as the inverse of the predicted probability from a logistic model, in which the presence of a measure at time 3 was predicted by the time 2 pain score (linear trend term). For time 4, a similar procedure was used to give weights that varied with the time 3 pain score. These last could only be estimated where such a score was available and thus were conditional upon response at time 3. Thus observations eventually included in the analysis were: all time 1, all time 2, all available time 3 where each was weighted by a simple weight, and all available time 4 observations that also had time 3 observations and where each was weighted by the product of simple weights at time 3 and time 4. In the main analysis account is taken of the fact that these non-response weights are not frequency weights by the use of the robust covariance estimator.

Results of the three analyses are compared in Table 7.14. The fitted models all indicate a significant and large negative main effect for time, reflecting a marked reduction in severity over time in the comparison group. The negative estimate for the interaction with

Table 7.14. Longitudinal Proportional Odds Model for Pain Data of Table 7.13.

Variable	Missing Value Method	Log-odds Estimate	95% Confidence Interval
Treatment			
	AAO	0.688	(−0.684, 2.060)
	Weighted	0.720	(−0.702, 2.142)
	LOCF	0.562	(−0.806, 1.929)
Time			
	AAO	−1.197	(−1.670, −0.723)
	Weighted	−1.164	(−1.668, −0.660)
	LOCF	−1.156	(−1.608, −0.703)
Treatment by time			
	AAO	−0.242	(0.849, 0.365)
	Weighted	−0.264	(−0.911, 0.382)
	LOCF	−0.181	(−0.706, 0.344)

AAO = All Available Observations,
Weighted = inverse probability weighting,
LOCF = Last Observation Carried Forward.

treatment is consistent with treatment leading to a slightly quicker recovery, but the effect is not significant and the confidence intervals are wide. Thus the substantial differences in the point estimates arising from the different treatments of missing data do not alter the overall pattern of inference (though the unjustified narrowing of the confidence intervals using LOCF is apparent — see Chapter 5).

The analysis undertaken in constructing the weights, in fact, corresponds to a model of non-response. The models examined here made use of the immediately prior pain score as the only predictor. For both time 3 and time 4, the direction of effect was such that those with more severe pain were more likely to return for treatment, but in neither case was the association significant ($p = 0.6$ and 0.3, respectively). The response models could have included treatment or any other available variable. Although in many circumstances there can be a range of different response models that yield weights that give largely comparable results, differences can arise and the scope for discretion in the choice of weighting model can be large. Particular care needs to be taken where any observations are associated with unusually large weights. In this example, the final weights for time 4 observations ranged from 1.26 (observation 14) to 2.21 (observations 9 and 17).

7.7. SUMMARY

This chapter has outlined and illustrated the three main approaches to the analysis of non-normal longitudinal data: the marginal approach; the random effects or mixed modelling approach; and the transition model approach. Though less unified than the methods available for normal data, these methods provide powerful and flexible tools to analyse, what until relatively recently, have been seen as almost intractable data. However, as with any such tool, care in their use is required.

The random effects and transition models approaches, being based on probability models, can be estimated by maximum likelihood. This gives them a capability with respect to dealing with data missing at random. Use of the weighting method described in this chapter, however, extends the marginal approach to circumstances where missing data may not be missing completely at random.

CHAPTER 8

Survival Analysis

8.1. INTRODUCTION

In many clinical trials, the main response variable is often the time to the occurrence of a particular event. In a cancer study, for example, surgery, radiation and chemotherapy might be compared with respect to the time from randomisation and the start of therapy until death. In this case the event of interest is the death of a patient, but in other situations it might be the end of a period spent in remission from a disease, relief from symptoms, or the recurrence of a particular condition. Such data are generally referred to by the generic term *survival data* even when the endpoint or event being studied is not death but something else. Questions of interest for such data involve comparisons of survival times for different treatment groups and the identification of prognostic factors useful for predicting survival times. Since these do not differ from the questions usually posed about other response variables used in clinical trials, it might be asked why survival times merit any special consideration, in particular a separate chapter? There are a number of reasons. The first is that survival data are generally not symmetrically distributed — they will often be positively skewed, so assuming a normal distribution will not be reasonable. A more important reason for giving survival data special treatment is the frequent occurrence in such data of *censored observations*. These arise because at the completion of the study, some patients may not have reached the endpoint of interest (death, relapse, etc.). Consequently, their exact survival times are not known. All that *is* known is that the survival times are *greater* than the amount of time the patient has been in the study. This is *right-censoring*. A further reason for the special attention paid to survival times is that measuring time is conceptually different from measuring other quantities.

The analysis of survival data from clinical trials will be covered relatively concisely in this chapter. Fuller accounts of survival analysis are available in Kalbfleisch and Prentice (1980), Cox and Oakes (1984), Lee (1992) and Collett (1994). In this chapter, the notation that we have used is the traditional one. In Chapter 9 we illustrate the counting process notation that is growing in favour.

8.2. THE SURVIVOR FUNCTION AND THE HAZARD FUNCTION

The analysis of a set of survival data from a clinical trial usually begins with a numerical or graphical summary of the survival times for individuals in the different treatment groups. Such summaries may be of interest in their own right, or as a precursor to a more detailed analysis of the data. Two functions describing the distribution of survival times which are of central importance in the analysis of survival data are the *survivor function* and the *hazard function*.

8.2.1. Survivor Function

The survivor function, $S(t)$ is defined as the probability that the survival time, T, is greater than or equal to t, i.e.,

$$S(t) = \Pr(T > t) \tag{8.1}$$

If the random variable T has a probability density function $f(t)$, then the survivor function is given by:

$$S(t) = \int_t^\infty f(u)du = 1 - F(t), \tag{8.2}$$

where $F(t)$ is the cumulative distribution function of T.

Two probability distributions often used to introduce the analysis of survival data are the *exponential distribution* and the *Weibull distribution*. The probability density function of the former is:

$$f(t) = \lambda e^{-\lambda t} \quad t \geq 0, \quad \lambda \geq 0 \tag{8.3}$$

and of the latter:

$$f(t) = \lambda \gamma t^{\gamma-1} \exp[-\lambda t^{\gamma}] \quad t \geq 0, \quad \gamma, \lambda > 0 \tag{8.4}$$

This is a Weibull distribution with scale parameter λ and slope parameter γ. (The exponential distribution is a special case of the Weibull distribution with $\gamma = 1$.)

Examples of each density function for a variety of parameter values are shown in Fig. 8.1

The survivor function for the exponential distribution is:

$$S(t) = \int_{t}^{\infty} \lambda e^{-\lambda u} du = e^{-\lambda t}, \tag{8.5}$$

and for the Weibull distribution

$$S(t) = \int_{t}^{\infty} \lambda \gamma u^{\gamma-1} \exp[-\lambda u^{\gamma}] du = \exp[-\lambda t^{\gamma}] \tag{8.6}$$

Graphs of these survivor functions for various parameter values are shown in Fig. 8.2.

Estimation of such parametric models is commonly approached using maximum likelihood, where for individual i, the likelihood has the form

$$L_i(\boldsymbol{\theta}) = f(t_i|\boldsymbol{\theta})^{d_i} S(t_i|\boldsymbol{\theta})^{1-d_i} \tag{8.7}$$

where d_i is an indicator variable for death/failure ($1 = $ death, $0 = $ censored) and $\boldsymbol{\theta}$ is the parameter vector of the distribution. In the case of the simple exponential model, the ML estimate of the single parameter λ reduces to the observed sample total of failures divided by the total follow-up time.

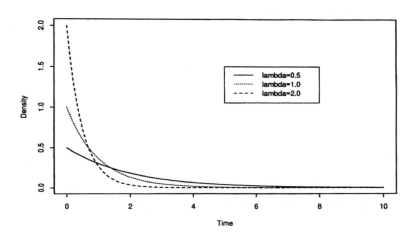

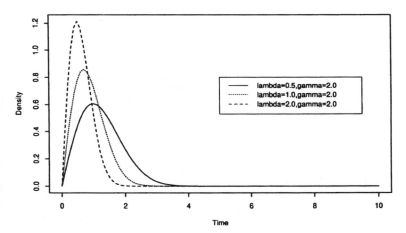

Fig. 8.1. Weibull and exponential density functions.

Where there are no censored observations in the sample of survival times, a nonparametric survivor function can be estimated simply as:

$$\hat{S}(t) = \frac{\text{number of individuals with survival times} \geq t}{\text{number of individuals in the data set}} \quad (8.8)$$

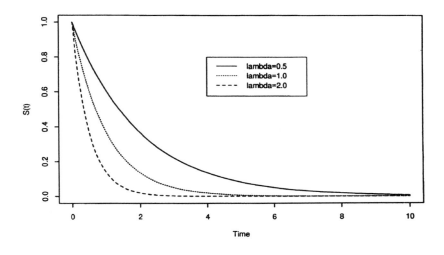

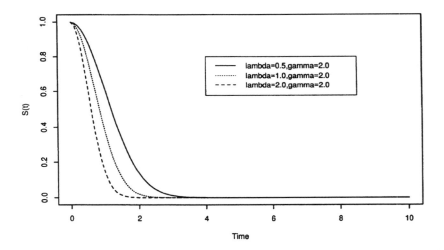

Fig. 8.2. Survivor functions for exponential and Weibull distributions.

(This is a nonparametric estimator since no particular distribution is assumed.)

The estimated survivor function is assumed to be constant between two adjacent death times, so a plot of $\hat{S}(t)$ against t is a step-function. The function decreases immediately after each observed survival time.

The simple method of estimating the survivor function described by Eq. (8.8) can only be used if all the individuals are followed up until the particular event of interest has happened to each. A number of methods are available for estimating the survivor function for survival data containing censored observations. That most commonly used is the *Kaplan–Meier* or *product limit estimator*. This involves first ordering the survival times from the smallest to the largest such that $t_{(1)} \leq t_{(2)} \leq \cdots \leq t_{(n)}$, and then applying the following formula to obtain the required estimate:

$$\hat{S}(t) = \prod_{j|t_{(j)} \leq t} \left(1 - \frac{d_j}{r_j}\right) \tag{8.9}$$

where r_j is the number of individuals at risk just before $t_{(j)}$, and d_j is the number who experience the event of interest at $t_{(j)}$ (individuals censored at $t_{(j)}$ are included in r_j). The variance of the Kaplan–Meier estimator is give by:

$$\text{Var}[\hat{S}(t)] = [\hat{S}(t)]^2 \sum_{j|t_{(j)} \leq t} \frac{d_j}{r_j(r_j - d_j)} \tag{8.10}$$

We shall illustrate the use of the Kaplan–Meier estimator on the data shown in Table 8.1. These data arise from a randomised controlled clinical trial to compare two treatments for prostate cancer. The treatments were a placebo and 1.0 mg of diethylstilbestrol (DES). The treatments were administered daily by mouth and the trial was double blind. The survival times of the 38 patients are given in months. We are interested in determining whether there is any evidence of a treatment difference in survival.

The estimated survivor functions of the two groups are shown in Fig. 8.3. Since the distribution of survival times tends to be positively skewed, the median is usually the chosen measure of location. Once the survivor function has been estimated, it is generally

Table 8.1. Survival Times of Prostatic Cancer Patients in Clinical Trial to Compare Two Treatments.

ID	Treatment	Survival	Status
1	1	65	0
2	2	61	0
3	2	60	0
4	1	58	0
5	2	51	0
6	1	51	0
7	1	14	1
8	1	43	0
9	2	16	0
10	1	52	0
11	1	59	0
12	2	55	0
13	2	68	0
14	2	51	0
15	1	2	0
16	1	67	0
17	2	66	0
18	2	66	0
19	2	28	0
20	2	50	1
21	1	69	1
22	1	67	0
23	2	65	0
24	1	24	0
25	2	45	0
26	2	64	0
27	1	61	0
28	1	26	1

Table 8.1. (*Continued*)

ID	Treatment	Survival	Status
29	1	42	1
30	2	57	0
31	2	70	0
32	2	5	0
33	2	54	0
34	1	36	1
35	2	70	0
36	2	67	0
37	1	23	0
38	1	62	0

Treatment: 1 = placebo, 2 = DES.
Status: 0 = censored, 1 = died.

straightforward to obtain an estimate of the *median survival time.* This is the time beyond which 50% of the individuals in the population of interest are expected to survive.

Although examining plots of estimated survivor functions is a useful initial procedure for visually comparing the survival experience of different treatment groups in a clinical trial, we generally also wish to test formally for a difference in survival between the groups. In the absence of censored observations, standard nonparametric or parametric tests might be used. When the data contain censored observations, however, there are a number of modified parametric and nonparametric tests that are available. Here we shall consider only one, namely the *log-rank* or *Mantel–Haenszel test.* Essentially this test compares the observed number of deaths occurring at each particular time point with the number to be expected if the survival experience of the two treatment groups was the same. A small numerical example of the application of the test to hypothetical data is described in Table 8.2.

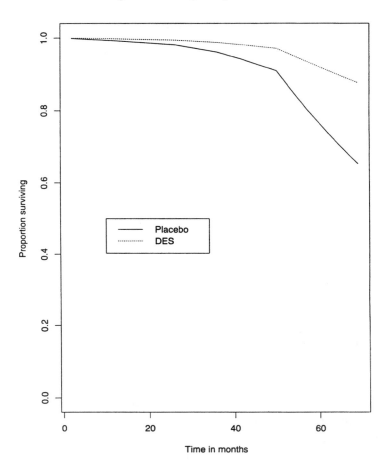

Fig. 8.3. Kaplan-Meier estimated survivor functions for the two treatment groups in the prostate cancer trial.

For the prostate trial data we have:

Group	n	Observed	Expected	$(O-E)^2/E$
Placebo	18	5	2.475	2.577
DES	20	1	3.525	1.809

Table 8.2. Calculation of Log-Rank Test for a Hypothetical Set of Survival Times in Two Groups.

Survival times

Patient	Treatment	Survival time	Status
1	1	2.3	dead
2	1	4.8	alive
3	1	6.1	dead
4	1	15.2	dead
5	1	23.8	alive
6	2	1.6	dead
7	2	3.8	dead
8	2	14.3	alive
9	2	18.7	dead
10	2	36.3	alive

Calculating log-rank test

Time

1.6		T1	T2	Total
	Dead	0(0.5)	1(0.5)	1
	Alive	5	4	9
	Total	5	5	10

2.3		T1	T2	Total
	Dead	1(0.55)	0(0.45)	1
	Alive	4	4	8
	Total	5	4	9

3.8		T1	T2	Total
	Dead	0(0.5)	1(0.5)	1
	Alive	4	3	7
	Total	4	4	8

Table 8.2 (*Continued*)

Calculating log-rank test

Time		T1	T2	Total
6.1				
	Dead	1(0.5)	0(0.5)	1
	Alive	2	3	5
	Total	3	3	6
15.2		T1	T2	Total
	Dead	1(0.5)	0(0.5)	1
	Alive	1	2	3
	Total	2	2	4
18.7		T1	T2	Total
	Dead	0(0.33)	1(0.67)	1
	Alive	1	1	2
	Total	1	2	3

Expected number of deaths are shown in parentheses. 'Alive' means alive *and* at risk.

Observed number of deaths for T1 = 3;
Expected number of deaths for T1 = 0.5 + 0.55 + 0.5 + 0.5 + 0.5 + 0.33 = 2.89.

Observed number of deaths for T2 = 3;
Expected number of deaths for T2 = 0.5 + 0.45 + 0.5 + 0.5 + 0.5 + 0.67 = 3.11.

$$X^2 = \frac{(3 - 2.89)^2}{2.89} + \frac{(3 - 3.11)^2}{3.11} = 0.008$$

This leads to a chi-squared value of 4.4 with a single degree of freedom. The associated p-value is 0.0355 and there is evidence of a difference in the survival experience of the two treatment groups. Patients given DES appear to survive longer. The simple conceptual construction of this score test has considerable appeal, one that is valuable in communicating results to non-expert audiences.

8.2.2. The Hazard Function

In the analysis of survival data it is often of some interest to assess which periods have the highest and which the lowest chance of death (or whatever the event of interest happens to be), amongst those people alive at the time. In the very old, for example, there is a high risk of dying each year, among those entering that stage of their life. The probability of any individual dying in their 100th year is, however, small because so few individuals live to be 100 years old.

A suitable approach to assessing such risks is to use the *hazard function*, $h(t)$, defined as the probability that an individual experiences an event (death, relapse etc.) in a small time interval s, given that the individual has survived up to the beginning of the interval, i.e.,

$$h(t) = \lim_{s \to 0} \frac{\Pr(\text{event in } t, t+s)}{s} \qquad (8.11)$$

The hazard function is also known as the *intensity function, instantaneous failure rate* and the *age specific failure rate*.

The hazard function can also be defined in terms of the cumulative distribution and probability density function of the survival times as:

$$h(t) = \frac{f(t)}{1 - F(t)} = \frac{f(t)}{S(t)} \qquad (8.12)$$

It then follows that:

$$h(t) = -\frac{d}{dt}\{\ln S(t)\} \qquad (8.13)$$

and so

$$S(t) = \exp\{-H(t)\} \qquad (8.14)$$

where $H(t)$, the *integrated* or *cumulative hazard function* is given by:

$$H(t) = \int_0^t h(u)\, du \qquad (8.15)$$

For the exponential distribution, the hazard function is simply λ; for the Weibull distribution, it is $\lambda\gamma t^{\gamma-1}$. The Weibull can accomodate increasing, decreasing and constant hazard functions.

The hazard function can be estimated as the proportion of individuals experiencing the event of interest in an interval per unit time, given that they have survived to the beginning of the interval, i.e.,

$$\hat{h}(t) = \frac{\text{number of individuals experiencing an even in the interval beginning at time } t}{(\text{number of patients surving at } t)(\text{interval width})}$$

(8.16)

The sampling variation in the estimate of the hazard function within each interval is usually considerable. Plots of the cumulative hazard function, obtained by summing the interval estimates over time, are typically smoother and easier to interpret.

In practice the hazard function may increase, decrease, remain constant, or indicate a more complicated process. The hazard function for death in human beings, for example, has the 'bath tub' shape shown in Figure 8.4. It is relatively high immediately after birth, declines rapidly in the early years and then remains approximately constant before beginning to rise again during late middle age.

8.3. REGRESSION MODELS FOR SURVIVAL DATA

The log-rank test described in Section 8.2.1 can be extended to the case where there are either more than two patient groups to be compared or where there are possible confounding factors that may be treated as strata. But the test, and other similar tests, are limited in their ability to fully describe and model the data. Consequently, more complex analyses of survival data are usually performed using some type of specialised regression model.

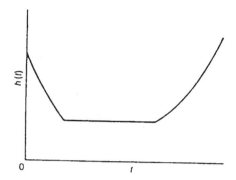

Fig. 8.4. Bathtub shaped hazard function.

The regression models that have been developed for survival data are essentially of two types. The first models the hazard function in patient groups compared to a baseline population by means of a multiplicative model, that is to say, additive on the log-hazard scale. The multiplicative factor is assumed to be constant over time, in which case the model forces the hazards in the different patient groups to be proportional, thus yielding a *proportional hazards regression model*. Following Peto (1976), estimates of the hazard ratio in the two sample case (A and B) can be obtained directly from the Mantel–Haenzsel log-rank test statistic and its variance (see Section 8.2.1). Alternatively, following Mantel and Haenzsel (1959), it may be estimated as:

$$\theta = \frac{\sum_{j=1}^{J} d_{A_j}(n_{B_j} - d_{B_j})/n_j}{\sum_{j=1}^{J} d_{B_j}(n_{A_j} - d_{A_j})/n_j} \tag{8.17}$$

The second type of regression model commonly applied to survival data, models the survival times directly, with covariates assumed to act multiplicatively directly on the time scale, thus accelerating or decelerating time to failure. The models are generally referred to as *accelerated failure time models*.

Within each of these two types of model, either the baseline hazard in the proportional hazards model, or the baseline survivor function in the acccelerated failure time model, can be assumed to be either fully parametric or modelled nonparametrically. Traditionally, however, proportional hazard models have been semi-parametric with the baseline hazard assumed nonparametric, and accelerated failure time models have been formulated as fully parametric.

8.4. ACCELERATED FAILURE TIME MODELS

The accelerated failure time model is a general model for survival data, in which covariates measured on an individual are assumed to act multiplicatively on the time-scale, and so can be thought of as influencing the rate at which an individual proceeds along the time axis. Such models can be interpreted in terms of the speed of progression of a disease. Algebraically, such models are of the form:

$$S_i(t) = S_0(\phi_i t) \tag{8.18}$$

where $\phi_i = \exp(\beta' \mathbf{x})$ is the *acceleration factor* for the ith patient compared with the baseline patient group.

The exponential and Weibull have already been introduced as possible survival distributions. Another distribution that is frequently used for survival data is the log-normal with density function:

$$f(t) = \frac{1}{\sigma\sqrt{2\pi}} t^{-1} \exp\{-[\ln(t) - \mu]^2 / 2\sigma^2\} \tag{8.19}$$

where μ is the mean and σ^2 is the variance. The log-normal distribution has a relatively heavy right tail, a feature that makes it useful for situations in which events occur later in the follow-up period.

The accelerated failure time model is most easily considered when it is expressed in log-linear form. Letting t_i denote the survival time for the ith subject, the model is:

$$\ln(t_i) = \beta_0 + \beta' \mathbf{x}_i + \sigma \epsilon_i \tag{8.20}$$

where σ is a scale parameter and ϵ_i assumed to have some suitable distribution. Gaussian errors and no censoring simply correspond to linear regression of log-survival time. More generally the model is used with distributions such as the exponential, Weibull, log-logistic, and gamma. It can be shown that if the errors are exponential or Weibull, then the model is also a proportional hazards model.

Parameter estimates can be found by maximising the likelihood function given by:

$$L(\theta) = \prod_{i=1}^{n} f(t_i)^{\delta_i} F(t_i)^{1-\delta_i} \qquad (8.21)$$

where $\theta' = [\beta_0, \beta, \sigma]$ and $\delta_i = 0$ if the event of interest has occurred, and $\delta_i = 1$ if the observation's survival time is censored.

We shall illustrate the application of the accelerated failure time model on the data from a randomised trial of chemotherapy for lung cancer (the data are given in Prentice, 1973, and Kalbfleisch and Prentice, 1980). The 137 patients, all but 19 of whom died during the trial, had survival times ranging from 1 to 999 days. In addition to standard and chemotherapy treatment, covariates included months since diagnosis, age, prior therapy, type of cancer (squamous, small, adeno and large) and the Karnofsky Performance Index of each patient's functional status that ranged from complete hospitalisation to normal self-caring.

The results under a number of different assumptions about the distribution of the survival times are given in Table 8.3.

The log-likelihoods under the three different distributional assumptions are very similar, being -196.75 for the exponential, -196.14 for the Weibull, and -195.22 for the log-normal. The exponential model has one less parameter than the other two, and represents a special case of the Weibull. A likelihood ratio test of the exponential against the Weibull gives: $\chi^2(1)$ of $2 \times (-196.14 - 196.75) = 1.22$, giving little evidence in favour of a systematically increasing or decreasing failure rate. The estimated Weibull parameter

Table 8.3. Results from Fitting Accelerated Failure Time Model to Survival Times from the Lung Cancer Trial.

Exponential

Covariate	Estimate	SE	Estimate/SE
Constant	2.59	0.75	3.45
Treatment	0.22	0.20	1.11
Months since DX	−0.01	0.01	−0.03
Karnofsky Performance Index/10	−0.31	0.05	6.00
Prior Treatment	−0.00	0.02	−0.21
Cell type:			
small v squamous	0.38	0.27	1.38
adeno v squamous	−0.44	0.26	−1.70
large v squamous	−0.74	0.29	−2.50
Log-L	−196.75		

Weibull

Covariate	Estimate	SE	Estimate/SE
Constant	2.64	0.71	3.72
Treatment	0.23	0.19	1.22
Months since DX	−0.00	0.00	−0.06
Karnofsky Performance Index/10	−0.30	0.05	6.23
Prior Treatment	−0.00	0.02	−0.20
Cell type:			
small v squamous	0.40	0.25	1.56
adeno v squamous	−0.43	0.24	−1.76
large v squamous	−0.74	0.27	−2.68
Scale	0.93		
Log-L	−196.14		

Table 8.3 (*Continued*)

Log-normal

Covariate	Estimate	SE	Estimate/SE
Constant	1.62	0.68	2.40
Treatment	0.17	0.19	0.89
Months since DX	−0.00	0.01	−0.13
Karnofsky Performance Index/10	−0.37	0.05	7.70
Prior Treatment	−0.01	0.02	−0.47
Cell type:			
small v squamous	−0.12	0.28	−0.42
adeno v squamous	−0.73	0.27	−2.71
large v squamous	−0.77	0.30	−2.59
Scale	1.06		
Log-L	−195.22		

is very close to 1, the value for a constant hazard. The log-normal model fits these data very slightly better than the Weibull.

Since all three models essentially fit the data equally well, it is not surprising that they give very similar estimates for the effects of covariates. Treatment is estimated as increasing the rate of progression along the time scale by $\exp(0.23) = 1.26$ or 26% under the Weibull model; and $\exp(0.17) = 1.19$ or 19% under the log-normal model, but confidence intervals are wide in both cases.

8.5. PROPORTIONAL HAZARDS MODEL

8.5.1. Proportional Hazards

A proportional hazards model possesses the property that different individuals have hazard functions that are proportional to one another, i.e., $h(t|\mathbf{x}_1)/h(t|\mathbf{x}_2)$, the ratio of hazard functions for two individuals with covariates $\mathbf{x}_1' = [x_{11}, x_{12}, \ldots, x_{1p}]$ and $\mathbf{x}_2' = [x_{21}, x_{22}, \ldots, x_{2p}]$, does not vary with time t. This implies that, given a set of covariates $\mathbf{x}$, the hazard function can be written as:

$$h(t|\mathbf{x}) = h_0(t)g(\mathbf{x}) \tag{8.22}$$

where $g(\mathbf{x})$ is a function of $\mathbf{x}$ and $h_0(t)$ can be regarded as a baseline hazard function for an individual for whom $g(\mathbf{x}) = 1$. The model forces the hazard ratio between two individuals to be constant over time since:

$$\frac{h(t|\mathbf{x}_1)}{h(t|\mathbf{x}_2)} = \frac{g(\mathbf{x}_1)}{g(\mathbf{x}_2)} \tag{8.23}$$

If the relative risk function g is taken as the exponential, additive effects on the log-linear scale are obtained. The effects of covariates are such that the baseline hazard function, $h_0(t)$, is modified multiplicatively by covariates (including group indicators), so that the hazard function for an individual patient is:

$$h(t|\mathbf{x}) = h_0(t)\exp[\boldsymbol{\beta}'\mathbf{x}] \tag{8.24}$$

8.5.2.   The Semi-Parametric Proportional Hazard or Cox Model

Although specifying a parametric form for $h_0(t)$ is straightforward, such a modelling approach has been rendered largely obsolete since Cox (1972) proposed a model and estimation method that allowed the form of the baseline hazard to be left unspecified. The model is *semi-parametric* in the sense that only the relative risk part is modelled parametrically.

The parameter vector $\boldsymbol{\beta}$ is estimated by maximising a partial likelihood. Brief details are given in Table 8.4. Interest usually centres on the estimated regression coefficients rather than the baseline hazard. However, an estimate of the baseline hazard function can be obtained by a maximum likelihood approach suggested by Kalbfleisch

Table 8.4. Parameter Estimation in Cox's Regression Model.

- Assume first that there are no tied survival times and that $t_1 < t_2 < \cdots < t_k$ represent the k distinct times to the event of interest among n individual times.

- The conditional probability that an individual with covariate vector $\mathbf{x}_i$ responds at time t_i, given that a single response occurs at time t_i, and given the risk set R_i (indices of individuals at risk just prior to t_i), is the ratio of the hazards:

$$\frac{\exp(\boldsymbol{\beta}'\mathbf{x}_i)}{\displaystyle\sum_{j \in R_i} \exp(\boldsymbol{\beta}'\mathbf{x}_j)}$$

- Multiplying these probabilities together for each of the k distinct survival times gives the following partial likelihood function (Cox, 1975):

$$L(\boldsymbol{\beta}) = \prod_{i=1}^{k} \frac{\exp(\boldsymbol{\beta}'\mathbf{x}_i)}{\displaystyle\sum_{j \in R_i} \exp(\boldsymbol{\beta}'\mathbf{x}_j)}$$

- Notice that the partial likelihood is a function of $\boldsymbol{\beta}$ only — it does not depend on the baseline hazard $h_0(t)$.

- Maximisation of the partial likelihood function yields estimates of the regression coefficients with properties similar to those of usual maximum likelihood estimators.

- When there are ties amongst the survival times, the likelihood function used for estimation is usually that proposed by Breslow (1974):

$$L(\boldsymbol{\beta}) = \left\{ \prod_{i=1}^{k} \frac{\exp(\boldsymbol{\beta}'\mathbf{s}_i)}{\left[\displaystyle\sum_{j \in R_i} \exp(\boldsymbol{\beta}'\mathbf{x}_j) \right]_i^{m}} \right\}$$

where m_i is the number of events at t_i and s_i is the vector sum of the covariates of the m_i individuals with survival time t_i.

and Prentice (1973). In the particular case where there are no tied survival times the estimated baseline hazard function at time $t_{(j)}$ is given by:

$$\hat{h}_0(t_{(i)}) = 1 - \hat{\lambda}_i \tag{8.25}$$

where

$$\hat{\lambda}_i = \left(1 - \frac{\exp(\hat{\beta}'\mathbf{x}_{(i)})}{\displaystyle\sum_{j \in R(t_{(i)})} \exp(\hat{\beta}'\mathbf{x}_{(i)})^{\exp(-\hat{\beta}'\mathbf{x}_{(i)})}}\right) \tag{8.26}$$

where $\mathbf{x}_{(i)}$ is the vector of explanatory variables for the individual who experiences the event of interest at time $t_{(i)}$. (Since the baseline hazard function is the hazard function for an individual having zero values for all the explanatory variables, it is often helpful to redefine variables by subtracting average values over all individuals in the sample.)

The baseline survivor function can now be estimated from:

$$\hat{S}_0(t) = \prod_{j=1}^{k} \hat{\lambda}_j \tag{8.27}$$

for $t_{(k)} \le t \le t_{(k+1)}, k = 1, 2, \ldots, r - 1$. The estimated value of the baseline survivor function is zero for $t \ge t_{(r)}$ unless there are censored survival times greater than $T_{(r)}$, in which case it is undefined beyond $t_{(r)}$. From $\hat{S}_o(t)$, the estimated survivor function for the ith individual with vector of covariates $\mathbf{x}_i$ is:

$$\hat{S}_i(t) = [\hat{S}_o(t)]^{\exp(\hat{\beta}'\mathbf{x}_i)} \tag{8.28}$$

The structure of the model as a regression model becomes easier to see if we rewrite the model as specified in Eq. (8.24) as:

$$\ln\left\{\frac{h(t)}{h_0(t)}\right\} = \beta'\mathbf{x} \tag{8.29}$$

showing that the proportional hazards model may also be regarded as a linear model for the logarithm of the hazard ratio. Consequently, the estimated regression coefficient corresponding to a particular covariate gives the change in the logarithm of the hazard function produced by a unit change in the variable, conditional on the other covariates remaining constant.

The variance of the regression coefficients derived from maximum partial likelihood are typically obtained in the conventional way from the inverse of the negative matrix of second derivatives of the log-partial-likelihood. But, as in the case of logistic regression, an exponential transformation of the coefficients is often preferred, giving more interpretable hazard ratios. However, the hazard ratio scale typically gives a likelihood function that is not quadratic and estimates that are not normally distributed. As a consequence, both Wald test p-values and confidence intervals perform poorly if directly calculated using a variance–covariance matrix on this scale. Instead, these are generally derived from the estimates and covariance matrix on the log-linear coefficient scale, confidence intervals being based on exponential transformation of the corresponding end-points of the log-linear interval.

We have seen from Chapter 4 that an alternative parameter variance–covariance estimator is the sandwich estimator based on the score residuals. The use of this estimator has been proposed in the survival context by Lin and Wei (1989). For generalised linear models (Chapter 4), this estimator is particularly valuable for clustered data, a feature that is implicit within the Cox model in which the same individual can appear repeatedly as a member of a series of risk sets (see Table 8.4). This reoccurrence of the same individual within the likelihood is emphasised on recognising that the likelihood treats equivalently data deriving from one individual who contributes to two risk sets, and data in which that individual is replaced in the second risk set by another individual with identical covariate values.

8.5.3. Cox Model Example

To illustrate the use of Cox's proportional hazards model, we use the data from the lung cancer trial. For simplicity, we consider only two of the explanatory variables. These are treatment and the Karnofsky Performance Index, a continuous score that was a powerful predictor of survival. We have previously followed others in fitting this index in its raw form, but given the exponential inverse link of proportional hazards models it might be more natural to fit the model to the log-transformed index. Indeed, the model does fit slightly better using the log-index rather than the raw index. The log-hazard ratio estimates for this model are given in Table 8.5. Again, there is no evidence of a treatment effect.

It is of interest to compare the width of the confidence intervals from this model with those from a parametric model. Fitting the corresponding Weibull model gave a confidence interval for the treatment effect of width 0.694 on the log-hazard ratio scale, compared to a width of 0.714 from the Cox model of Table 8.5. It is clear that there is little loss in the precision of the estimates of interest in using a non-parametric baseline hazard.

The estimates of Table 8.5 are for coefficients on the log-linear scale rather than the more easily interpreted hazard ratio scale. Following the previous section, and taking as an example the estimated coefficient for treatment conditional upon the Log-Performance Index given in Table 8.5, the hazard rate for patients treated with chemotherapy is $\exp(0.0637) = 1.066$ times the hazard rate for patients given the placebo. The corresponding 95% confidence interval is $(0.75, 1.52)$. The inclusion of the value one within this interval is consistent with no evidence of a treatment effect (positive or negative). Variation in response to this treatment depending upon the

Table 8.5. Cox Proportional Hazards Model Estimates: Lung Cancer Trial Data.

	Log-Haz. Ratio	Std. Err.	z	p-value
Treatment	0.064	0.182	0.35	0.7
Log-Performance Index	-1.424	0.200	-7.13	< 0.001

Table 8.6. Comparison of Standard (S), Robust (R) and Weighted (W) Estimates for Lung Cancer Trial Data.

	Haz. Ratio	Std. Err.	z	p-value	95% Conf. Interval
Treatment					
Standard	1.066	.194	0.349	0.73	(0.75, 1.52)
Robust	1.066	.203	0.334	0.74	(0.73, 1.55)
Weighted	1.077	.181	0.441	0.66	(0.77, 1.50)
Log-Performance Index					
Standard	0.241	.048	−7.132	< 0.001	(0.16, 0.36)
Robust	0.241	.064	−5.358	< 0.001	(0.14, 0.41)
Weighted	.312	.084	−4.304	< 0.001	(0.18, 0.53)

type of tissue affected would not be surprising. Though not shown, it is of interest to note that the inclusion of an interaction between treatment and cell-type shows marginal significance, consistent with squamous types being more responsive to this chemotherapy treatment than other types.

Table 8.6 presents the hazard ratios and 95% confidence intervals for effects of treatment and Performance Index. In addition, it also presents confidence intervals and p-values based on the sandwich estimator of the parameter covariance matrix. These are a little larger than the corresponding values using the conventional information matrix approach We defer discussion of the weighted estimator shown in the table to Section 8.5.6.

The estimated baseline survivor function for the lung trial data are shown in Table 8.7 for selected failure times. As a result of the prior standardisation of the explanatory variables about their mean values, this corresponds to the survivor function when all the covariates (including treatment group) are at their mean values. We can use the values in Table 8.7 to calculate the estimated survivor functions for the standard and chemotherapy ($68/137 = 0.496$ of the sample) treatment groups when the other covariates are at their

Table 8.7. Estimated Baseline Survivor Function at Selected Intervals for Lung Cancer Trial Data.

Survival time	Survival Prob. Standard Treatment	Survival Prob. Standard and Chemotherapy
1	1.0000	0.9782
125	0.3532	0.2267
249	0.1261	0.1017
373	0.0540	0.0525
497	0.0094	0.0177
621	.	0.0095
745	.	0.0095
869	.	0.0095
993	.	0.0027
1117	.	.

average values as follows:

$$\text{survivor function standard treatment} = [\hat{S}_0(t)]^{\exp[-1.066(0-0.496)]}$$

$$(8.30)$$

$$\text{survivor function chemotherapy} = [\hat{S}_0(t)]^{\exp[-1.066(1-0.496)]}$$

$$(8.31)$$

Plots of the estimated survivor functions are shown in Fig. 8.5.

8.5.4. Checking the Specification of a Cox Model

Cox's regression model makes two key assumptions:

- The effect of covariates is additive and linear on a log-hazard scale.

This linearity assumption is similar to that found in most other modelling methods we have considered in previous chapters.

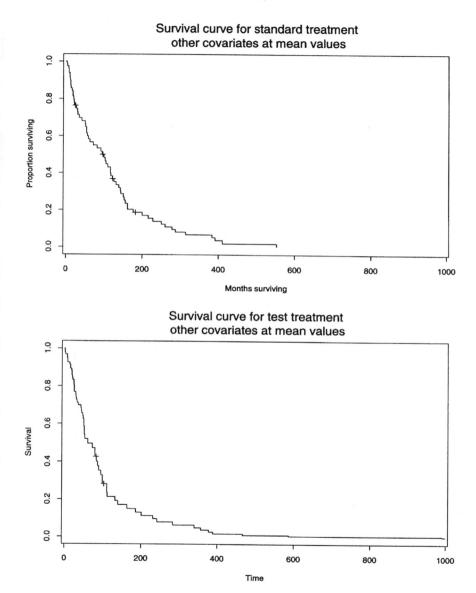

Fig. 8.5. Estimated survivor functions for the two treatment groups in the lung cancer trial when other covariates are fixed at their mean values.

- The ratio of the hazards of two individuals is the same at all times.

The proportionality assumption applies to all regressors in the model and not just the treatment effect, and a lack of proportionality can arise for a variety of reasons:

(1) Non-instantaneous treatment benefit. A treatment may require some time to be implemented following the randomisation time point or may require several sessions to become effective. Some treatments may carry short term risks which it is hoped are compensated by longer term benefits. Surgical treatments typically are of this kind, with complications leading to initial excess mortality when compared to a nonsurgical treatment.

(2) The effect 'wears off' over time. The treatment might halt disease progression but only temporarily or the disease may become progressively insensitive to the treatment as the treatment period is extended.

(3) A predictor variable may be time varying but the model represents its effect as due to a single baseline measure. As time goes on, the baseline measure comes to reflect the contemporaneous value of the covariate less and less well and thus becomes less predictive of subsequent survival. For the treatment variable, this can arise through a 'drift' away from the treatment protocol, e.g., as a result of increasing non- and poor compliance by patients or inadequate monitoring. For covariate effects such as measures of disease severity, individual variation in the progression of the disease will mean that severity at baseline no longer reflects current severity.

(4) Baseline measures are measured subject to error at the time of measurement.

(5) Effects are not uniform across patients. This might arise where the treatment benefit applies only to a subsample of individuals, such that over time those for whom treatment has no effect are lost from the treated sample.

To an extent, the particular tests and checks that one might use of the modelling assumptions and the extensions of the model that might be considered, will depend upon which of these possible causes of nonproportionality are suspected.

As in the checking of other models, residuals play a key role. A number of different residuals have been proposed for the Cox model.

- *Cox–Snell residual*; this is defined for the ith individual as:

$$r_{Ci} = \exp(\hat{\beta}'\mathbf{x}_i)\hat{H}_0(t_i) \qquad (8.32)$$

where $\hat{H}_0(t_i)$ is the estimated cumulative baseline hazard function at time t_i, the observed survival time of the individual. If the model is correct, then r_{Ci} will follow an exponential distribution with mean one, regardless of the actual distributional form of $S(t_i)$.

- *Martingale residual*; this is formed by taking the difference between the event indicator, δ_i and the Cox–Snell residual:

$$r_{Mi} = \delta_i - r_{Ci} \qquad (8.33)$$

Such residuals can be used to assess whether any particular patients are poorly predicted by the model, with large negative or positive residuals indicating a lack of fit. They can also be used together with continuous covariates for assessing the functional form required for the covariate with a random scatter about zero, indicating that the variable does not need transforming.

- *Deviance residual*; this may be calculated from the martingale residual as follows:

$$r_{Di} = \text{sign}(r_{Mi}\sqrt{-2[r_{Mi} + \delta_i \ln(\delta_i - r_{Mi})]}) \qquad (8.34)$$

Such residuals are particularly useful in identifying individuals who are poorly predicted by the model, such individuals being indicated by large negative or positive values of r_{Di}.

• *Schoenfeld or Efficient Score Residuals*

Schoenfeld (1982) suggested the use of residuals derived directly from the score function of the partial likelihood. A set of partial scores for each event can be obtained using:

$$\hat{r}_j = U(\hat{\beta}) = \frac{x_j - \sum_{i \in R_j}[x_i \exp(\beta x_i)]}{\sum_{i \in R_j} \exp(\beta x_i)} \tag{8.35}$$

These compare the x vector of the subject who fails with its expected value among all those subjects at risk. For each regressor, one (partial) residual is obtained for each event, a feature as we show below that is convenient for checking for homogeneity of effect over the course of a trial.

Using once again the lung cancer trial data, Fig. 8.6 shows the martingale residuals from the fitted Cox's regression model plotted

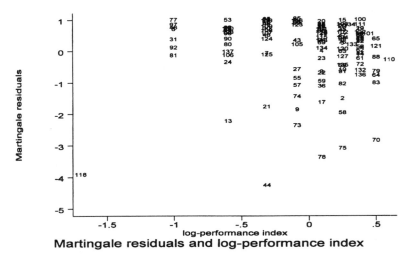

Martingale residuals and log-performance index

Fig. 8.6. Martingale residuals from the Cox's regression model fitted to the survival times from the lung cancer trial potted against the continuous covariate.

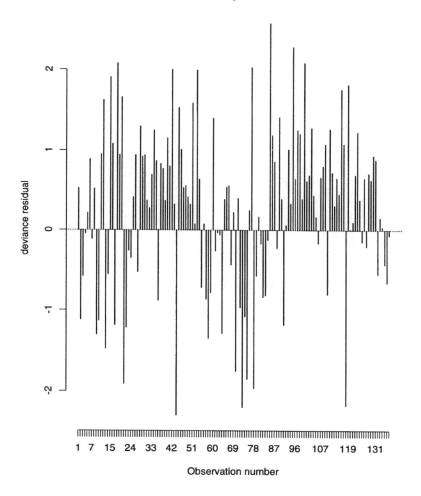

Fig. 8.7. Index plot of deviance residuals from Cox's regression model fitted to the survival times from the lung cancer trial.

against the continuous covariate log-Performance Index. Figure 8.7 is an index plot of the deviance residuals. The most obvious feature of all the plots is the consistently large value associated with patient 118 (who had unusually low performance at the start of the trial, having an index value of just 10), and to a lesser extent patient

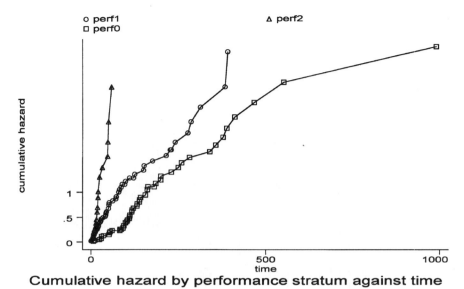

Cumulative hazard by performance stratum against time

Fig. 8.8. Cumulative hazard functions for strata defined by the Karnofsky Performance Index from the lung cancer trial.

44 (who survived an unusually long time given their relative poor performance index value of 40).

Numerous graphical plots have been proposed for checking the proportionality assumption (see Chen and Wang, 1991). Such plots should have a clear and simple pattern when the proportionality assumption holds. Plots of the cumulative hazard by sub-groups, each with a particular covariate pattern, are an obvious possibility, but this typically requires a course grouping of patients. We grouped patients from the lung cancer trial into three categories of the Performance Index. Figure 8.8 shows the three empirical cumulative hazard functions. These should form straight lines from the origin, but in this case are not fully convincing.

Alternatively, a double logarithmic transformation of Eq. (8.23) gives:

$$\ln[-\ln(S(t))] = \beta x + \ln[-\ln(S_o(t))] \qquad (8.36)$$

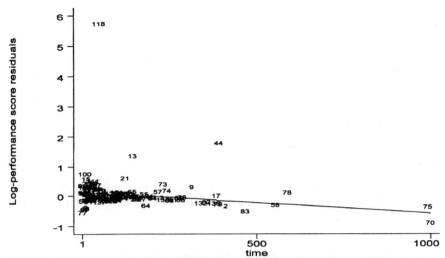

Scatter and smooth of score residuals for log-performance

Fig. 8.9. Schoenfeld (1982) or partial score residuals and regression smooth plotted against log-Karnofsky Performance Index from the lung cancer trial.

Thus, plots of the empirical log cumulative hazards for subgroups based on shared covariate patterns should, when plotted against t, appear parallel.

The partial score residuals introduced earlier should form a horizontal line when plotted against time or the failure rank. The addition of a regression smooth to the plot aids interpretation. The slope shown in Fig. 8.9 is suggestive of nonproportionalty.

In practice, however, it is quite often difficult to assess these plots and they can sometimes be misleading (Crowley and Storer, 1983). Thus, in addition to graphical checks, some formal specification testing is also desirable.

Cox (1972) suggested testing for time-variation in proportionality of effects of a variable z by the incorporation of a time-dependent variable $z* = z \cdot g(t)$. Common choices for the function $g(t)$ are

$g(t) = t$, $g(t) = \ln(t)$ and a step function such that $g(t) = 0$ if $t < T$ and 1 if $t \geq T$. We describe and illustrate how such time-varying variables can be included in Section 8.6. A likelihood ratio test can be performed of the models with and without the time-varying co-variate, or the coefficient for the time-dependent variable can be compared with its standard error for a Wald test. O'Quigley and Pessione (1989) proposed a score test for departures from nonpro-portionality of a similar structure. All these tests potentially involve some arbitrary choice of the alternative, and quite often this choice has been based on some preliminary inspection of the data, a prac-tice which needs to be taken into account when interpreting results (notably nominal p-values).

Gill and Schumacher (1987) suggested a test based on a compar-ison between two hazard ratio estimators, that differ in the relative weight that they assign to early versus late failures, in particular the Mantel–Haenszel (see Section 8.5.1) and Prentice estimators. If the hazards are really proportional, changes in weighting should have little effect. For groups A and B, a hazard ratio estimator is:

$$\hat{\theta} = \frac{\sum_{j=1}^{J} w_j \hat{\lambda}_{A_j}}{\sum_{j=1}^{J} w_j \hat{\lambda}_{B_j}} \tag{8.37}$$

For the the MH estimator, the weights w_j are given by $\frac{n_{A_j} n_{B_j}}{n_j}$, and for the Prentice estimator, by $\frac{n_{A_j} n_{B_j}}{n_j} \prod_{k=1}^{j} \frac{n_k - d_k + 1}{n_k + 1}$.

8.5.5. Goodness-of-fit Tests

As we have seen earlier the log-rank (MH) test is a score test that compares the observed number of deaths in groups of patients with those expected under a model of equal hazards. The tests of Schoen-feld (1980) and Moreau *et al.* (1986) can be thought of as an extension of such an approach in which firstly, the groups to be compared represent not just a partitioning of the covariate space (patient groups) but also of the time axis, and secondly, the expected deaths are derived from the fitted Cox model. Crouchley and Pickles (1993) describe a general class of specification test that is easily estimated from residuals, for both focussed hypotheses and for more general omnibus tests. Although probably superior to the use of graphical methods, simulations showed that the simple method for constructing the omnibus test tended to reject too often, suggesting specification errors where none in fact were present.

8.5.6. Influence

In the standard design of trial, the construction of the partial likelihood means that as survival time increases, so the risk set becomes smaller. Thus individuals with the longest survival time contribute not only through their numerous appearances in the risk sets prior to their failure/censoring, but also to those risk sets near the end of the trial in which few subjects are being compared. As a result, individuals with the longest survival are most likely to be influential points.

One simple approach to ensure that estimates are robust to the possible presence of such individuals, is to artificially censor all observations at some earlier point in the trial. This can be considered an extreme form of a weighted partial likelihood in which likelihood contributions beyond the artificial censoring time are given a weight of 0. More systematically, Sasieni (1993) suggests that the contribution to the partial likelihood of each risk set be weighted by a quantity proportional to the total number of individuals still at risk. The Kaplan–Meier survivor function suggests itself as one such possible quantity. The inclusion of such weights requires the use of the 'robust' estimator of the parameter covariance matrix.

We illustrate in Table 8.6 the use of Kaplan–Meier weighting for the lung cancer trial data. In this instance, the weights make very little difference to the estimated treatment effect, but the hazard ratio effect estimate for the log-Performance Index has moved closer to the null value of one. The inclusion of the weights has also increased the size of the standard error, reducing the corresponding z-statistic. The results again cast some doubt on the model specification with respect to this powerful prognostic factor.

In other respects, the influence of data points and the analysis of influence can be approached in a similar fashion to that described in Chapter 4 for generalised linear models. Thus subjects with covariate measurements that are extreme in the space of covariate values should be carefully checked. The score residuals described earlier are equivalent except for standardisation to the empirical influence function (Cain and Lange, 1984; Reid and Crepeau, 1985). Deletion diagnostics can be pursued in the usual way (Storer and Crepeau, 1985).

8.6. TIME-VARYING COVARIATES

8.6.1. Modelling with Time-Varying Covariates

Trials often include covariates with values that do not remain fixed over time. It is tempting, therefore, to consider making allowance for the changes in such variables by taking repeated measures of them during the operation of the trial and by fitting a model that uses these updated covariate values. In fact, this is simply done, merely requiring the survival period of each patient to be divided up into a sequence of shorter survival spells, each characterised by an entry time and an exit time, and within which covariate values remain fixed. Thus the data for each patient is represented by a number of shorter censored spells and possibly one spell ending in failure/death. Datasets can be constructed in exactly this form, each record representing one spell and containing, an entry time, an exit time, and a censoring indicator together with the then current covariate values. With multiple spells per patient, the file thus contains multiple records per patient.

Time-varying covariates are especially tractable within the Cox model. Inspection of Table 8.4 shows how the partial likelihood involves contributions for the conditional probability of failure. These conditional probabilities involve the covariate values that apply at the time of each failure only. The values of the covariates between failure times do not enter the partial likelihood. All that is required is that contemporaneous rather than baseline values of covariates be assigned to each risk set, making the Cox model with time-varying covariates little more complex than that for time-fixed covariates. Indeed for covariates that change rapidly over time the Cox model is often simpler to manage than a parametric survival model.

For illustration we divided the follow-up of the lung-cancer patients into two periods, before and after 75 days, that each contained approximately 50% of the deaths. Patients with follow-up times fewer than 75 days contributed just their original record. The remaining patients contributed one record with a censored survival time at day 75, then a second record with their original follow-up time and outcome but with entry into the trial given as day 75. A dummy variable is constructed to distinguish between the two follow-up periods. Fitting a model with an interaction between period and treatment or period and covariate provides a test of the constant proportionality of effect that the Cox model assumes. In this case, fitting the interaction between period and log-Performance Index gave a z-test with $p = 0.035$, casting some doubt on the assumption. In the first period, the hazard ratio was estimated at 0.20, while for second it was 0.69. This is not an uncommon pattern for a baseline measure, the prognostic value being rather short-lived.

8.6.2. The Problem of Internal or Endogeneous Covariates

Although simply incorporated into proportional hazard survival models, the use of time-varying covariates in analysis of clinical trials data should be approached with some caution. This is because their inclusion runs the risk of biasing the treatment effect as a result of their being internal, i.e., they reflect the development of the disease process and may themselves be partly influenced by treatment. Biochemical or physical measures of disease are obvious examples. This is well illustrated in the example of Altman and DeStavola (1994). High levels of bilirubin and low levels of albumin reflect advanced biliary cirrhosis and are highly prognostic. A treatment that improves cirrhosis will tend to reduce bilirubin levels and increase those of albumin. Altman and DeStavola showed how much of the significant and substantial estimate of treatment effect could be removed by the inclusion into the model of updated values of either of these variables. From the point of view of treatment effect estimation, updating these variables is most unwise, casting unnecesary doubt on treatment differences. From the point of view of a scientific investigation of the development of the process and for constructing prognostic indices, their inclusion will be of more interest.

Thus, it is important that internal or endogeneous variables should be distinguished from external or exogeneous variables. External variables are either predeterminded, e.g., a patients age, or vary independently of survival, e.g., the weather. However, for many time varying variables their status as internal or external is uncertain, which explains our caution. It is perhaps most helpful to think of internal variables as being those that are 'causally downstream' of treatment, but the link between treatment and variable does not have to be a direct one. Thus if the poor health of those on the worse or placebo treatment results in their choosing to move to a more pleasant and health promoting climate, then not even the weather is external!

8.6.3. Treatment Waiting Times

One circumstance where the use of time-varying covariates may be helpful is where the timing of the delivery of one or both treatments is not under complete experimental control. Such circumstances frequently arise in organ and tissue transplantation, where at the time of randomisation, no suitably well matched donors may be available for all patients. Two comparisons then become of interest. The first essentially defines the treatment as that given, i.e., a waiting time of unknown duration followed by transplantation, and compares survival over both waiting and post-transplant survival periods combined. The second defines the treatment as transplantation for which only the post-transplant survival is relevant. These correspond to the two rather different clinical circumstances of considering the treatment alternatives of a patient for whom a well matched donor is already available (the second case) and a patient for whom one is yet to be found (the first case). Without a very rigorous protocol, it is often unreasonable to assume that the waiting time to find a well-matched donor is independent of transplant survival, since matching criteria are likely to be relaxed as the waiting time increases and transplantation may only be possible if the patient is fit enough to survive surgery.

8.7. STRATIFICATION, MATCHING AND CLUSTER SAMPLING

8.7.1. Stratification

We have already seen how non-proportionality may be addressed by generalising the model by the addition of a function of the suspect predictor variable as a time dependent covariate. However, this approach requires that the functional form describing the pattern of time variation be specified (e.g., a linear trend). Where the variable for which the proportionality assumption is in question is a categorical variable, then a more general approach is possible using stratification. Dividing the subjects into strata g, we specify a hazard of the form:

$$h(t|\mathbf{x}, g) = h_{0g}(t) \exp(\boldsymbol{\beta}\mathbf{x}) \tag{8.38}$$

in which the effects for the covariate vector $\mathbf{x}$ (now shortened by the omission of the stratum identifying variable g) remain assumed to be proportional, but the baseline hazard is now quite separately estimated for each stratum. The contribution to the partial likelihood from each failure event is modified such that the risk set over which the denominator is calculated, is no longer all those at risk at that time, but only the subset of those who belong to the same stratum as the failing individual.

In practice, stratification is used to achieve a variety of goals:

(1) It can be applied to groups who either *a priori* may have quite different survival patterns, e.g., for example men and women, or *post-hoc* to groups defined by a variable that has failed a test of proportionality.

(2) It can be applied so as to obtain distinct estimates of survivor, hazard or integrated hazard functions for the groups in question that are adjusted for the remaining covariates but which are otherwise unconstrained. Plots of the group specific functions can be used to check proportionality. This has particular appeal where the grouping variable is treatment as it provides a simple graphical illustration of possible variation in treatment effect over time.

(3) The grouping variable need not be a fixed grouping factor but may be time varying, e.g., a variable defining the state of the disease. Strata can also be defined to distinguish between the different durations, e.g., first event, second event and so on in a recurrent event process.

8.7.2. Matching

Where patients have been matched, the simplest approach to analyse the resulting data is to specify each matched group as a separate stratum. For a simple two-treatment trial, the resulting partial likelihood corresponds to conditional logistic regression with contributions only from strata in which the first of the time ranked survival times in a pair is a failure time (i.e., pairs in which either the shortest time or both times in a pair are censored make no contribution).

8.7.3. Cluster Sampling

An alternative approach is to ignore the clustering in model estimation but to take account of it in the estimation of the parameter covariance matrix by using a robust estimator. It should be emphasised that these two approaches estimate slightly different parameters, the first being conditional upon any effects associated with the matching variables and the second being the effect marginal to/averaging over them.

Segal and Neuhaus (1993) exploit the fact that the survival likelihood can be formulated as a Poisson likelihood and can thus be made amenable to the Generalised Estimating Equations approach to GLM estimation described in Chapter 4. The likelihood in such a formulation for individual i in cluster j is of the form:

$$\mu_{ij}^{d_{ij}} \exp(-\mu_{ij}) \frac{h_o(t)}{H_o(t)^{d_{ij}}} \tag{8.39}$$

where $h_o(t)$ and $H_o(t)$ are the baseline hazard and integrated hazard, respectively, and the Poisson rate parameter μ_{ij} is specified by a log-linear model of the form:

$$\ln \mu_{ij} = \ln H_o(t) + \beta' \mathbf{x}. \tag{8.40}$$

The term $\ln H_o(t)$ in this last equation can be an offset, specified as $\ln(t)$ if the model is exponential or the Breslow estimate of $H_o(t)$ if the model is a Cox model (requiring iterative updating), or it can be estimated, for example, as a set of dummy variables defined for segments of the follow-up time to give a piecewise exponential model. GEE estimation of the model parameters and of the correlation among individual survival times of individuals from the same cluster j then follows in the usual way as described in Chapter 6.

Yet another approach to clustered data treats the correlation in survival times as deriving from the hazard (or log-hazard) containing a shared random effect. This is discussed in Sections 8.10 and 9.5.

8.8. CENSORING AND COMPETING RISKS

The discussion so far has given rather little consideration as to how censored observations may have come about. Indeed, because they seem to pose no practical difficulty for analysis, it is far too easy to give them inadequate consideration. Clearly censored observations coincident with a data-independent end of a trial pose no special source of concern, but this may not be the case for losses to follow-up occurring during the process of the trial. Losses may occur through patient noncompliance or inadequacies in the implementation of the trial. These raise all the issues and concerns relating to missing data, discussed in previous chapters. In other circumstances, losses may be disguised as failures, the result of some parallel survival process that cannot be suppressed during the period of the trial. Death from other causes than the focal cause is the typical example. On the assumption that this other process is conditionally independent of the process of interest, then these failures from other causes can be treated as providing censored observations from the process of interest.

Table 8.8 compares the Cox model estimates and standard errors for the effects of age, surgery and mismatch score on survival following heart-transplant for an all-causes outcome and for an outcome

Table 8.8. Estimated Effects of Prognostic Indicators — Stanford Heart Transplant Data.

Model/Effect	Hazard Ratio	z	95% Confidence Interval
Death — All Causes			
log(age in years)	14.64	2.28	(1.45, 147.44)
log(mismatch score)	4.27	1.95	(0.99, 18.36)
Death — Rejection only			
log(age in years)	422.78	3.24	(10.89, 16333)
log(mismatch score)	17.71	3.05	(1.79, 112.63)

restricted to death from rejection (all other outcomes contributing censored observations). The data come from the much analysed Stanford Heart Transplant programme (Crowley and Hu, 1997). The increased estimate and significance for the effect of quality of transplant match, when nonrejection related failures are excluded, is striking.

The potential impact of reclassifying outcomes as defined by the censoring indicator is thus considerable and the example serves to underscore the need for careful prior thought being given to the measurement protocol and for the importance of maintaining blindness through to the end of trial measurement (and perhaps even beyond, into the analysis stage).

8.9. AUXILIARY VARIABLES

Where a variable is clearly endogeneous, although we might not wish to include it as an independent variable within our analysis, we might be able to increase the power of our analysis by considering it as informative about the end-point of the trial. For example, some endogeneous biological marker might be used to define an intermediate state of disease progression within what would now be a multi-state survival model. This would have the effect of reducing the number of fully censored observations. Treatment effects on the risk functions to both the intermediate state and the final end state can then be estimated, using the framework of competing risks described in the previous section. Hsieh *et al.* (1983) and Pocock *et al.* (1987) consider the analysis of two time-dependent events. However, as our previous discussion of multiple end-points in Chapter 4 made clear, the question of how to combine effects requires assigning some measure of relative importance to them. This has not always proved straightforward.

An alternative is to assume that the importance of the event is reflected in its effect on the final end-point itself. Lagakos (1977) described an approach for using auxiliary information for this purpose within a simple exponential survival framework. Finkelstein and

Schoenfeld (1994) present a method that uses the time to the intermediate state as a covariate for subsequent survival. Their simulations suggest that although improvements in precision of the estimates of main interest are possible, losses of efficiency are also possible where the intermediate state is not strongly prognostic. The use of weighted estimating equations provides one of a number of other approaches to this problem (Robins and Rotnitsky, 1992).

8.10. FRAILTY MODELS

One of the ways in which it was suggested that non-proportionality might come about was in a context in which individuals varied in their risk of death in ways not reflected in the included covariates. This lack of homogeneity has been conceptualised as implying the presence of a random effect in the hazard function and has been termed frailty. The sharing of frailty may also be a useful way of considering the correlation in response of patients that have been formed into matched groups similar on a set of prognostically relevant variables, sampled by a multi-stage process (e.g. individuals within families) or the correlations among repeated or multivariate survival times that might arise from experimental response time measurements. A number of authors have investigated the impact of frailty on estimated effects (e.g., Chastang *et al.*, 1988; Pickles and Crouchley, 1995) and this can be large for endogeneous variables. This issue also relates to the possible presence of long-term survivors or cured individuals (Farewell, 1982). Pickles and Crouchley (1994) also considered models in which dose-response was a random effect. Such models can now be relatively easily fitted using multilevel modelling software (Goldstein, 1991). We illustrate in Chapter 9 the Bayesian estimation of a frailty model for the matched pairs data.

It is very tempting to interpret the hazard function as saying something about the development of risk within the individual. A decreasing hazard rate is often interpreted as expressing a biological phenomenon associated with the individual in which (s)he becomes in some way stronger, more robust or less vulnerable. Unfortunately, the hazard rate is not a pure measure of within subject variation. High risk or frail individuals will tend to have short survival times, resulting in a selection over time for those who were more robust from the outset. This selection causes the usual estimated hazard rate to decline, or to rise less rapidly. The inclusion of frailty within the model can be used in an attempt to account for these selection effects.

8.11. INTERIM ANALYSIS FOR SURVIVAL TIME DATA

Interim analysis has been discussed in Chapter 3. The reasons given there for its use apply equally well to trials in which the main response variable is time-to-death, time-to-relapse, etc. Tsiatis (1981) demonstrates a number of important results that show the distributional structure of the log-rank test, computed over time, is similar to that for instantaneous outcome measures, allowing the theory developed for such measures to be used in the more complex survival analysis setting. For details, readers are referred to the two papers mentioned and the EaSt manual (see Appendix). Here, we simply give an example.

8.11.1. An Example of the Application of an Interim Analysis Procedure for Survival Data

DeMets and Lan (1994) describe the use of group sequential methods in a randomised, double-blind, placebo-controlled trial designed to test the effect of propranolol, a beta blocker drug, on total mortality. In a multicentre recruitment, 3837 patients were randomised between propranolol or placebo. The study used the log-rank test for comparison of the survival patterns of the two groups and adopted the group sequential boundaries suggested by O'Brien and Fleming. Seven interim analyses were planned and the relevant O'Brien–Fleming boundaries are shown in Fig. 8.10. The results of the log-rank test are

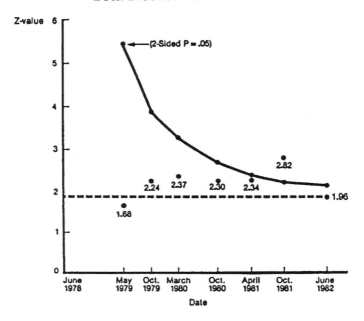

Fig. 8.10. O'Brien and Fleming boundary for log-rank test in a randomised double blind trial.

also shown as the trial progressed. On the 5th interim analysis, the log-rank test approached but did not exceed, the critical value. On the 6th interim analysis, the logrank statistic was 2.82 and exceeded the critical value of 2.23. This resulted in stopping of the trial almost a year earlier than planned.

8.12. DESCRIBING THE RESULTS OF A SURVIVAL ANALYSIS OF A CLINICAL TRIAL

A number of measures of effect for survival and lifetime data have been suggested that may help communicate results to different audiences. The absolute risk reduction (ARR) is given by the difference in survival probabilities for the two treatments, for some suitable choice of time t, ARR $= S_{A(t)} - S_{B(t)}$. Using the Kaplan–Meier estimates for $S(t)$, a variance for the ARR can be obtained as

$$\text{var}(\text{ARR}) = [1 - \hat{S}_{A(t)}][\hat{S}_{A(t)}]^2/n_{A(t)} + [1 - \hat{S}_{B(t)}][\hat{S}_{B(t)}]^2/n_{B(t)}$$
(8.41)

where $n(t)$ is the size of the risk set at time t. The ARR can be made more concrete by multiplying by the size of the treatment arm of the trial to give a number of deaths avoided (NDA $=$ ARR $\times n$), with a variance given by n times var(ARR). It is sometimes suggested that the estimated number of patients in the population who might benefit from the treatment be used in this calculation to give an estimate of the therapeutic impact. Care is required here, in that the size may be rather poorly known and it is in general unlikely that the characteristics of this wider group of patients will be like those enrolled in the trial.

An increasingly common measure is the number needed to treat (NNT), the inverse of the absolute risk reduction (NNT $= 1/$ARR). Like the ARR, this must be reported together with the length of follow-up that is being assumed. A confidence interval can be obtained by inverting the corresponding endpoints of the interval for the ARR.

Epidemiologists find the risk ratio RR a natural scale. Given by $(1 - S_{A(t)})/(1 - S_{B(t)})$, it allows effects to be described in terms of a halving (or some other fraction) of the risk. Note that it, too, requires specifying the relevant follow-up period. An estimate of its variance can be obtained using Fieller's theorem (see Marubini and Valsecchi, 1995). A relative risk reduction or difference, $1 - RR(t)$, is also sometimes used.

8.13. SUMMARY

Survival analysis is the study of the distribution of times to some terminating event (death, relapse etc.). A distinguishing feature of survival data is the presence of censored observations and this has led to the development of a wide range of methodology for analysing survival times. Of the available methods, the most widely used is Cox's proportional hazards model which allows the investigation of the effects of multiple covariates on the hazard function. The model has been almost universally adopted by statisticians and applied researchers particularly for survival times arising from a clinical trial. But other models for survival data are also available and one of these, the accelerated failure time model, is also described in this chapter.

Whatever the particular form of survival model chosen, a number of common issues arise, principally in the area of model checking. Although less well developed than for continuous response measures, various methods for model checking are available. These include model generalisations, residuals, plots and goodness-of-fit and specification tests. However, in a number of instances these methods do not work well as a reliable diagnostic for *overall* correct model specification. Instead, testing of survival models works best when the statistician has some idea of the likely alternative models. In such circumstances, it is understandable why statisticians so frequently resort to the use of the Cox survival model, since its nonparametric baseline hazard leaves one less aspect of the model to check, and little loss of efficiency is incurred when compared to parametric models. Nonproportionality can often be addressed by the careful use of strata, time-varying variables are readily included, and extensions to competing risks by redefinition of the censoring indicator is straightforward.

CHAPTER 9

Bayesian Methods

9.1. INTRODUCTION

Until relatively recently, Bayesian statistics were little more than an intellectual curiousity; rich in conceptual insight but of little practical value when it came to actual data analysis. All this has changed in the most dramatic fashion, with Bayesian methods and applications now forming an area of the most intense activity. In many cases, Bayesian approaches lead to the same or similar conclusions as those using the routine procedures of the frequentist statistician. But differences do occur and there are proponents on each side with, for example, Berry (1993) presenting the case for greater use of Bayesian methods in clinical trials and Whitehead (1993) presenting the case for the ongoing dominance of the frequentist approach, at least in the context of definitive phase III trials. Most statisticians involved in trials are typically rather pragmatic, for the most part using the familiar and quick to apply frequentist methods, but nonetheless also applying Bayesian methods where these are convenient or have some conceptual advantage and are acceptable to the intended consumer. Much recent work proposing Bayesian methods in clinical trials has been concerned as much with establishing acceptability as with developing the methods.

Traditional frequentist analysis essentially treats each trial or experiment as if it were entirely novel and each trial is usually being considered as being individually potentially decisive. Scientific progress may occur outside the narrow focus of this trial, but the numerical procedures themselves are not formulated to reflect the process of progressive learning nor one in which the process itself involves costs and potential benefits. By contrast, the focus of Bayesian methods is one of progressive refinement of opinion as data from trials and other sources accumulate. This is illustrated in Fig. 9.1. Knowledge prior to a trial is synthesised and formally represented as a distribution over the parameter space of the problem. The trial is undertaken. The data from the trial is combined with the prior distribution to form a posterior distribution over the same parameter space, one which is hopefully more concentrated than the prior.

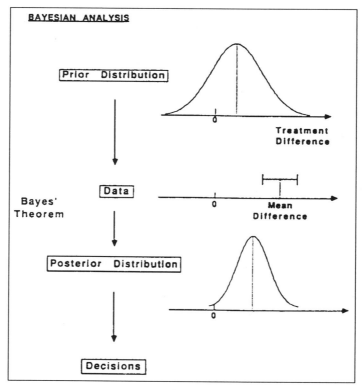

Fig. 9.1. Conceptual framework for Bayesian analysis.

While this may describe well the circumstances of the developers of a treatment, who will be building up knowledge about a treatment through various phases of the development and trialling process, licensing authorities have typically been comfortable with the frequentist position, the results from a phase-III trial, complete with all its formal rigours, being key to their decision making. Nonetheless, even in the context of phase-III trials, Bayesian methods can provide valuable additional insights, particularly in relation to considerations of sample size requirements and interim analyses.

As described above, the focus of Bayesian methods is on using data to update prior beliefs, as defined by parameter or effect distributions. If one starts from a position of diffuse and uninformative prior distributions, then the focus of the analysis is little different from that of other methods. As a result, non-Bayesian's are increasingly making use of the recent developments in Bayesian model estimation. We therefore start with a brief description of Bayesian estimation, before considering other more distinctive aspects of Bayesian inference for clinical trials.

9.2. BAYESIAN ESTIMATION

From a Bayesian perspective, both observed data and parameters are considered as random quantities. Letting D denote the observed data and Θ the model parameters, a joint probability distribution or *full probability model* $P(D, \Theta)$ is considered, which is decomposed into a *prior distribution* for the parameters $P(\Theta)$ and a *likelihood* $P(D|\Theta)$ for which:

$$P(D, \Theta) = P(D|\Theta)P(\Theta) \qquad (9.1)$$

Given data from a trial, the *posterior distribution* of the parameters Θ, that is the distribution of Θ given the data, is obtained by use of Bayes' Theorem,

$$P(\Theta|D) = P(\Theta)P(D|\Theta)/ \int P(\Theta)P(D|\Theta)d\Theta \qquad (9.2)$$

Quantities calculated from this posterior distribution of the parameters form the basis of inference. Point estimates might be obtained by calculating the mean, mode or median of a parameter posterior distribution, while the parameter precision can be estimated by the standard deviation or some suitable inter-quantile range, e.g., from quantiles at p and $1 - p$ for a $100(1 - 2p)\%$ credible interval. In general such quantities, $f(\Theta)$, will be estimated by their posterior expectation given by:

$$E[f(\Theta)|D] = \int f(\Theta)P(\Theta)P(D|\Theta)d\Theta \Big/ \int P(\Theta)P(D|\Theta)d\Theta \quad (9.3)$$

As an illustration of the mathematics of Bayesian inference, consider a sequence of Bernoulli trials. At the outset, we will assume that we can characterise any prior knowledge that we have as to the likely value of the Bernoulli probability θ in a prior distribution. It is mathematically convenient to choose a so-called conjugate distribution as the prior distribution for θ, which in this case is a beta distribution with density $b(p)$:

$$P(\theta) = \theta^{\alpha-1}(1 - \theta)^{\beta-1}\Gamma(\alpha + \beta)/\Gamma(\alpha)\Gamma(\beta) \quad (9.4)$$

This has mean $\alpha/(\alpha + \beta)$ and variance $\alpha\beta/((\alpha + \beta)^2(\alpha + \beta + 1))$. Figure 9.2 shows four beta distributions. Symmetrical unimodal distributions are obtained for $\alpha = \beta > 1$, narrowing as their value increases, becoming asymmetrical when α does not equal β. Also notice that although $\alpha = \beta = 1$ is uniform over θ, calculation of the variance shows that larger variances are obtained from bimodal shapes in which α and β tend to zero.

In a sequence of n trials we observe r successes, giving a likelihood $P(n, r|\theta)$ proportional to $\theta^r(1 - \theta)^{n-r}$. Equation 9.2 shows that the posterior distribution is obtained by multiplying the prior distribution by this likelihood and standardising. The selection of a conjugate prior makes this straightforward, giving

$$P(\theta|d, n) \propto \theta^{\alpha+r-1}(1 - \theta)^{\beta+n-r-1} \quad (9.5)$$

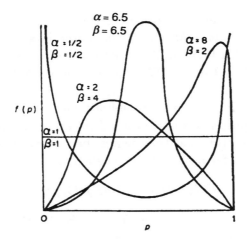

Fig. 9.2. Four beta distributions.

which is another beta distribution but with parameters $\alpha* = \alpha + r$ and $\beta* = \beta + n - r$.

The mean of this posterior distribution is $(\alpha + r)/(\alpha + \beta + n)$, with a corresponding expression to that given above for the variance. As a consequence as α and β approach zero, corresponding to a prior distribution with the greatest possible variance, so the posterior mean approaches r/n, the value that would be expected under maximum likelihood. As r and n increase relative to α and β, so the the variance of the distribution approaches the familiar $(r/n) \times (1 - (r/n))/n$.

Figure 9.2 shows a beta distribution with $\alpha = \beta = 6.5$, the posterior distribution that would occur following the observation of 6 successes in 12 trials with the use of the reasonably uninformative prior in which $\alpha = \beta = 0.5$ (also shown).

9.3. MARKOV CHAIN MONTE CARLO (MCMC)

In the hypothetical example of the previous section, the particular choice of likelihood and prior allowed the necessary expectations to be calculated by hand. In practice, this is not generally possible. Instead *Markov Chain Monte Carlo* methods are used; these are based on Monte-Carlo integration methods for tackling the numerical problems posed by Eq. 9.3. We give here only the briefest sketch of MCMC estimation.

Monte Carlo integration consists of a method for drawing values of Θ from the posterior distribution $P(\Theta|D)$, calculating the corresponding values $f(\Theta)$ and then using their average to approximate $E[f(\Theta|D)]$. Thus for a 'sample' of m such values of Θ:

$$E[f(\Theta)|D] \sim 1/m\Sigma f(\Theta_m|D) \qquad (9.6)$$

For many methods of sampling from $P(\Theta|D)$, this approximation can be made as accurate as required simpy by increasing the size of the 'sample' m. One of these methods is to sample from a suitable Markov Chain that has as its stationary distribution $P(\Theta|D)$, giving rise to the name of the overall estimation method.

One of the features of such a procedure is that, regardless of where it is started, in the long-run the state occupancy distribution tends to converge to the equilibrium stationary distribution. Thus the MCMC method consists of a 'burn-in' during which it is intended that the stationary distribution should be achieved, followed by a period of 'monitoring' during which 'sample' values of the quantities of interest $f(\Theta)$ are recorded and during which tests of convergence are undertaken (Gelman, 1996). Readers are referred elsewhere for the theoretical background and for further discussion of available sampling algorithms (e.g. Roberts, 1996).

9.4. ADVANTAGES OF THE MCMC APPROACH

Although the principles behind the MCMC estimation and inference are no more complex than those of more traditional methods, it is a computational intensive method to put into practice. Therefore, it is helpful to have clear what some of the potential advantages are before setting out to implement such an analysis.

9.4.1. Model Parametrisation and Scientific Inference

The effects reported as the results of any model estimation exercise, e.g., maximum likelihood, are typically presented in the form in which the statistical model has been parametrised for estimation. Only sometimes are estimates and confidence intervals translated into a more readily understood scale. An example of this is logistic regression where considerations as to the multivariate normality of the estimators leads to estimation of effects on the log-odds scale, even though for most clinical audiences it is the odds-ratio scale that is most readily interpreted. As a result, it is perhaps more often the case than most statisticians appreciate that the parameters and associated confidence intervals commonly estimated are not those of greatest scientific interest or clinical relevance. The parametrisation with desirable statistical properties is rarely that with desirable scientific properties and the effort in translating results from one to the other, for example using the delta method, often holds little appeal to the statistician. However, in MCMC estimation, the parametrisation Θ over which the Markov Chain is defined, does not constrain the list of quantities $f(\Theta)$ for which posterior distributions are monitored. Thus Θ can be chosen for its statistical and estimation properties, while the $f(\Theta)$ can be chosen for their scientific and clinical interest. The additional burden of adding into the MCMC sampling cycle a variety of functions of the parameters is rarely great.

As an example, consider a study involving three drug treatments A, B and C and a control treatment; a standard parametrisation would be a mean contrast for the effects of each drug relative to the common control group. However, we might wish to know what the probability is that the pair of drugs that perform best in some small trial actually contains the 'best' drug. This kind of information is extremely valuable in drug development, but is not readily calculated from knowledge of the point estimates and covariance matrix of the standard parameters. It is, however, an extremely simple task to monitor the ranks of the effects of each treatment from each MCMC sample, and to obtain an estimate of their distribution, confidence intervals and so on.

A second example, one that we illustrate later in this chapter, is the estimation of the *Number Needed to Treat* (NNT) effect measure together with its confidence interval. A variety of other effect scales might be contemplated and the discussion in Chapter 5 relating to the summary statistic approach is relevant here, both for pointing to aspects of the trial that may be of interest, but also in warning of the need to have agreed a single decision criterion prior to the study, whenever that is appropriate.

9.4.2. Missing Data

No new ideas or methods are required to extend MCMC estimation to problems with missing data. The missing observations are merely added to the parameter list, and like the original parameters, are sampled from their conditional distributions. Monitoring of the estimated missing data values can be helpful in assessing the plausability of a model. The approach can be extended to consider 'hypothetical data points', for example those in the future, allowing an exploration of an individual subject's prognosis (Berzuni, 1996)

9.4.3. Prior Distributions as a Numerical Device

Although frequentists, in particular, may feel uncomfortable about the imposition of informative priors on parameters, there are many circumstances where the imposition of such priors merely act to keep parameter estimates within feasible bounds. In more standard ML estimation, such problems often require the use of a variety of somewhat *ad-hoc* 'fix-ups' that substantially complicate function maximisation algorithms and present additional problems where convergence is at a boundary solution. Imposing a suitable prior can result in a better behaved estimation procedure.

9.4.4.   Alternative Models and Model Selection

A Bayesian approach has often also been distinctive in showing a willingness to consider a range of alternative models, and, for example, using so-called *Bayes factors* to choose between them. These factors provide a summary of the evidence given by the data D in favour of a model M_1 relative to another model M_0; they are defined as the ratio of the posterior to prior odds,

$$B_{10} = \frac{P(D|M_1)}{P(D|M_0)} \tag{9.7}$$

Twice the logarithm of B_{10} is on the same scale as the deviance and the likelihood ratio test statistic. The following scale is often useful for interpreting values of B_{10}:

$2\ln B_{10}$	Evidence for M_1
< 0	Negative (supports M_0)
0–2.2	Not worth more than a bare mention
2.2–6	Positive
6–10	Strong
> 10	Very strong

Sometimes 'robust' estimates are considered that attempt to make a combined inference from a weighted average of the parameter estimates from different models. Considering a range of alternative models is clearly valuable, but we are less convinced about the value of this combining of different estimates. For example, when considering models with and without a nuisance parameter (say the effects of a possible confounder), it seems unreasonable to consider the problem as a bimodal one — a mixture of null and alternative values — rather than using prior information on what the value of the nuisance parameter is likely to be.

9.5. A NUMERICAL EXAMPLE OF USING BAYESIAN ESTIMATION

To illustrate the use of a Bayesian estimation method for an essentially non-Bayesian analysis, we have turned to the classic data of Frierich *et al.* (1963) on 6MP and placebo treatment of 42 leukemia patients. These data are shown in Table 9.1. Though much analysed, the paired design of this study has typically been ignored. Spiegelhalter *et al.* (1996) use the program BUGS (Gilks *et al.* 1994; see Appendix) to estimate a Cox regression model (see Chapter 8) that includes a random effect for pairing.

Table 9.1. Pairwise-Matched Trial of Remissions in Acute Leukemia (Frierich *et al.*, 1963).

Survival Time (weeks)	Death	Treatment	Pair ID
		(+0.5 = 6-mercaptopurine)	
1	1	0.5	1
1	1	0.5	2
2	1	0.5	3
2	1	0.5	4
3	1	0.5	5
4	1	0.5	6
4	1	0.5	7
5	1	0.5	8
5	1	0.5	9
8	1	0.5	10
8	1	0.5	11
8	1	0.5	12
8	1	0.5	13
11	1	0.5	14
11	1	0.5	15
12	1	0.5	16
12	1	0.5	17
15	1	0.5	18

Table 9.1. (*Continued*)

Subject ID	Death	Treatment	Pair ID
17	1	0.5	19
22	1	0.5	20
23	1	0.5	21
6	1	−0.5	19
6	1	−0.5	18
6	1	−0.5	8
6	0	−0.5	1
7	1	−0.5	20
9	0	−0.5	6
10	1	−0.5	2
10	0	−0.5	10
11	0	−0.5	3
13	1	−0.5	14
16	1	−0.5	4
17	0	−0.5	11
19	0	−0.5	7
20	0	−0.5	9
22	1	−0.5	12
23	1	−0.5	16
25	0	−0.5	17
32	0	−0.5	5
32	0	−0.5	13
34	0	−0.5	15
35	0	−0.5	21

Using the counting process notation (Anderson and Gill, 1982), we observe the count of the number of failures up to time t, $N_i(t)$ which has the intensity process:

$$I_i(t)dt = E[dN_i(t)|F_{t_-}] \qquad (9.8)$$

where F_{t_-} represents the data on the process up to time t. This expectation corresponds to the probability of subject i failing in the interval $[t, t + dt)$. As $dt \to 0$ and assuming a proportional hazards model with time constant covariates and time constant random effect for each pair, the intensity takes the form:

$$I_i(t) = Y_i(t)\lambda_0(t) \exp(\beta' x + \mu_{j(i)}) \tag{9.9}$$

where $j(i)$ is the pair to which patient i belongs. In line with many of the random effects models described in Chapters 6 and 7, the distribution of the random effects can be assumed normal, implying in this case a log-normally distributed multiplicative effect on the intensity itself.

The parameters of the model, therefore, include the regression parameters β, the baseline intensity $\lambda_o(t)$, and the precision (1/variance) of the random effect distribution. Spiegelhalter *et al.* choose a normal prior with very low precision as an uninformative prior for β. For the baseline intensity, it is convenient to consider the increments between failures as having a log-normal prior. For the precision of the random effect distribution, a gamma prior is convenient.

Having specified the prior distributions and starting values for the parameters, parameter estimates can be obtained through the use of Gibbs sampling. This involves drawing values from the conditional distributions of each parameter, given the data and current values of the other parameters, taking each parameter in turn. This process can be shown to converge, such that after a suitable 'burn-in' period, typically of the order of several and often many hundreds of iterations, the distribution of the parameter vector remains the same from iteration to iteration.

At this point, the variation in the values of the parameters from iteration to iteration represents the variance (and covariance) in their estimates as a result of having a limited amount of data. With uninformative priors and a well behaved problem, this typically corresponds closely to the sample variance–covariance matrix of parameter estimates that might be obtained by direct maximum-likelihood. So, after the 'burn-in' period, the stream of sample values for the

Table 9.2. Comparison of Cox Model Estimates for Leukemia Trial Data.

	Partial Likelihood SAS PHREG	MCMC Without Pairwise Frailty	MCMC With Pairwise Frailty
Treatment effect	1.59 (0.43)	1.55 (0.43)	1.58 (0.43)
Random effect SD			0.16 (0.03–0.69)

parameters are monitored and stored, and the empirical mean, medians, variances, covariances, confidence-intervals and so on are estimated directly from these values. Clearly, the number of sample values upon which these are estimated must be large enough to keep the simulation sampling error small. For the calculation of some statistics, such as extreme confidence intervals based on the empirical distribution (rather than a variance estimate), the simulation sample may need to be large (in excess of 1000).

Table 9.2 presents results of standard maximum-likelihood fitting of this Cox model without a frailty effect, and those obtained using Gibbs sampling with and without the frailty random effect. The variation in the estimates of the fixed treatment effect have rather more to do with the assumptions being made within each method about the treatment of ties (see Chapter 8) than with the particular estimation method, but this variation is anyway small. The estimate of the precision of the random effects distribution is consistent with a random effect variance of only 0.03, suggesting that the pairings were not well matched or were matched on the basis of factors and covariates of little prognostic significance.

As described above, within the iterations of the sampling algorithm additional functions of the parameters and data can be calculated. We added a function to estimate NNT. The posterior mean for NNT was estimated as 2.51, with a standard deviation of 0.96 and 95% credible interval of $(1.46, 4.87)$.

9.6.   INFORMATIVE PRIORS

In the previous example the priors were essentially uninformative, chosen largely to keep parameters within a feasible space, and their presence within the analysis had very little influence on the eventual results. If, however, informative priors are to be considered, the statistician enters what is for many the rather unfamiliar territory relating to the characterisation of prior beliefs. It is often convenient, both conceptually and in practice, to consider this process as one of translating prior beliefs into a hypothetical dataset. This dataset then informs a design in the same way that a meta-analysis of previous findings can inform a proposed study (see Chapter 10).

The choice of information source for a prior depends on the purpose to which it is to be put. For example, where studies are being undertaken within the context of an ongoing research programme, it makes sense to analyse and interpret the results of new studies as part of an ongoing accumulation of knowledge. However, while use of previous trials is appropriate in the assessment of final results, Freedman, Spiegelhalter and Parmar (1994) suggest that such data should play a more minor role in monitoring a new trial if it is to provide independent confirmation. Freedman and Spiegelhalter (1983) describe methods which we describe in the next section for eliciting subjective opinion. Stewart and Parmar (1993) discuss issues in relation to using previous studies.

9.7.   PRIORS AND STOPPING RULES FOR TRIAL MONITORING

We have already described in Chapter 3, how for many large trials, trial monitoring and the use of interim analyses are now routine practice, required both for ethical and financial reasons. It was also noted how the Bayesian approach to sequential analysis helped avoid a number of the difficulties encountered by the frequentist approach to this problem. It therefore makes sense to develop the Bayesian argument within such a context.

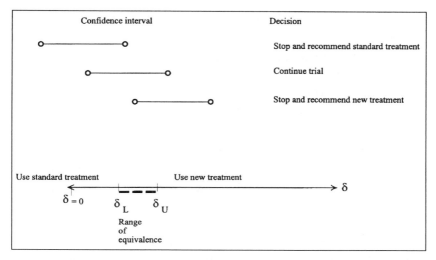

Fig. 9.3. Ranges of equivalence elicited from clinicians.

Freedman and Spiegelhalter (1983) proposed a framework for considering a new treatment versus a standard treatment. Two aspects of clinical opinion need to be considered: clinical demands and clinical beliefs.

9.7.1. Clinical Demands

Freedman and Spiegelhalter suggested that two levels of treatment improvement should be considered, as illustrated in Fig. 9.3. The lower value δ_L is the treatment effect below which a clinician would definitely not use the new treatment. It is referred to as the minimum clinically worthwhile difference. In this hypothetical case it is slightly positive, perhaps the result of the new treatment requiring new training, extra costs or patient discomfort. The upper value δ_U is the level of improvement above which the clinician would wish to switch to using the new treatment as routine. The range between δ_L and δ_U is referred to as the *range of equivalence*. As a study proceeds, decisions on continuing the trial are then made by comparing the confidence interval for the treatment effect with this range of equivalence. Where the confidence interval falls entirely above δ_L, the study should be stopped and the new treatment adopted as routine. Where the interval falls entirely below δ_U, the study should be stopped and the standard treatment continued as routine. If neither applies, then the trial should continue.

The values of δ_L and δ_U were obtained by interview with a range of clinicians involved in the treatment of the disease in question. Clinicians responded to the questions of the sort, "if the real benefit was $x\%$, would you use the new treatment as your routine?" Such questions were asked a number of times, changing the value of x up and down the scale, to identify the levels at which the clinician would definitely use (δ_U) and not use (δ_L) the new treatment. Such questioning yields results as illustrated in Fig. 9.4, with both the location and the width of the range of equivalence varying from clinician to clinician. The extent of overlap between the prior distribution and the range of equivalence provides the ethical basis for randomisation. Freedman and Spiegelhalter found considerable

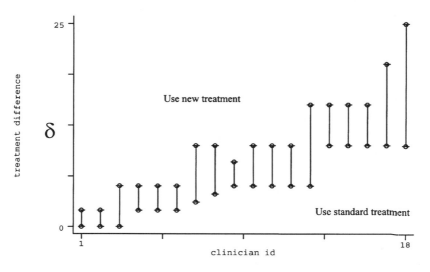

Fig. 9.4. Scheme for 'ethical' stopping rules for trial monitoring.

variation between clinicians in the elicited ranges of equivalence. This raised doubts as to the applicability of the simple decision rules described in the previous paragraph.

9.7.2.   Clinical Beliefs

In eliciting views on clinical beliefs clinicians were first asked what the 'most likely' level of improvement would be, then upper and lower bounds that were 'very unlikely to be exceeded' together with a judgement of what odds corresponded to 'very unlikely', and then similar questions for intermediate points. A sketch of this 'prior' was then verified and adjusted through discussion. There are, of course, a variety of other ways in which such distributions might be elicited. Parmar *et al.* (1994) present an example that makes use of analogue scales and the allocation of % beliefs over a set of ordinal categories. As in the case of clinical demands, substantial diversity of opinion was found, with marked between-clinician variation in location, dispersion and shape. As we will see, this heterogeneity of opinion, together with the fact that clinicians involved in a trial from whom priors are most likely to be sought and received, are likely to be enthusiasts for the new treatment, has prompted the consideration of a different approach to trial monitoring that we describe in a later section.

A summary of prior opinion can be formed from these individual assessments by approximating them by a fitted distribution. For survival data, a convenient scale on which to consider this issue is the log-hazard ratio, LHR, for which:

$$\exp(\text{LHR}) = \log(P_{\text{new}})/\log(P_{\text{standard}}) \qquad (9.10)$$

and P_{new} and P_{standard} are the survival rates (proportions) under the new and standard treatments, respectively. Assuming that the distribution on the log-hazard ratio is normally distributed, the prior can be characterised by a mean μ_0 and variance σ_0^2. Since for survival data (the Cox model) the variance is approximately equal to $4/n$, where n is the number of events (Tsiatis, 1981), the prior can be summarised by a mean μ_0 and an implicit number of events n_0.

9.8. MONITORING

9.8.1. The Prior as a Handicap

Subsequent real data arising out of the trial with which to update the prior are summarised by corresponding values μ_d and n_d. Combining the prior and data together using Bayes theorem gives a posterior mean μ_p, given by the simple weighted sum $(\mu_0 \times n_0 + \mu_d \times n_d)/(n_0 + n_d)$ with variance σ_p^2 given by $4/(n_0 + n_d)$. Undertaken early in the trial with little real data, the combined results will largely reflect the prior. Thus only the most extreme data could result in confidence intervals that did not include one or the other of the δ_L and δ_U, with correspondingly little chance of very early stopping of the trial. Undertaken late in the trial, the weight of data will dominate the influence of the prior, generating results that are similar to those of a traditional analysis. A typical prior thus acts as a *handicap*, restraining the study in the early phases from premature conclusions.

Grossman *et al.* (1994) provide a more structured approach for how the handicap can be used for interim analyses within a group sequential design. They consider a trial involving T sequential blocks, each of n/T patients, with analyses following the completion of each block. In addition, a handicapping prior sample of size $f \times n$, the size of f reflecting the extent of handicap desired, is included. Thus at the tth analysis, the sample size is $fn + nt/T$. If each block of patients has mean response Y_t, and the standard deviation of the response is σ, then the stopping rule test statistic is $Z_t = (Y_1 + Y_2 + \cdots + Y_T)\sqrt{(n/t_T)}/\sigma$. Without adjustment, the trial would stop if the test statistic exceeded the usual critical value Z_c, 1.96 in the case of $\alpha = 0.05$. Grossman *et al.* (1994) show how the inclusion of the handicap sample in a trial with t analyses increases the critical value of the test statistic by the factor $\sqrt{(t + fT)/t}$. Freedman, Spiegelhalter and Parmar (1994) compare this 'unified approach' to trial monitoring to the stopping rules of Pocock and of O'Brien and Fleming, and suggest the following handicap as fixing the Type I error rate at 5% for the specified number of analyses (given in brackets): 0.00 (1), 0.16 (2), 0.22 (3), 0.25 (4), 0.27 (5), 0.29 (6), 0.30 (7), 0.32 (8), 0.33 (9), and 0.33 (10).

9.8.2. Recognising Heterogeneity in Priors: Enthusiasts and Sceptics

The diversity of clinical opinion identified earlier suggests that searching for a decision rule based on the beliefs of some average or representative view may not be appropriate. An alternative basis for monitoring emphasises how different groups of clinicians interpret the results. This approach addresses the question of whether a typical sceptical clinician will be persuaded of the positive value of the new treatement and the complementary question as to whether a typical enthusiast will be persuaded of its inneffectiveness (see Spiegelhalter, Freedman and Parmar, 1994). A study should be aiming to do one or other of these. The prior of a typical enthusiast can be elicited from the participating clinicians using the techniques described above; it already being noted that involvement in a trial tends to select for clinical enthusiasm for the new treatment. The suggested prior of a typical sceptic is based on the experience in most fields that most new treatments have been found to be inneffective or at best only slightly better than the standard treatment. Such a prior is one centred on 0 with only 5% above the point of the alternative hypothesis (μ_0), i.e., a standard deviation σ_0 equal to the alternative hypothesis value divided by 1.645. This alternative value should be 'realistic' (not that often optimistically large value that is so often used in power calculations to justify the small size of a trial!). As with other priors, this can be conveniently thought of as a hypothetical dataset from a trial, in this case of N_0 patients, where N_0 is given by $2\sigma/\sigma_0$ with σ_0 as previously defined and σ the standard deviation of the response measure. The enthusiasts prior is then centred on δ with $\sigma = \sigma_0$.

Now, the usual sample size formula gives:

$$N = 4[z(1 - \alpha) + z(1 - \beta)]^2 \times \sigma^2/\delta^2 \qquad (9.11)$$

where α is the one-sided significance level, $1 - \beta$ is the power, δ is the alternative hypothesis and σ is the standard deviation of the response. But given that $\sigma_0 = \delta/z(1 - \gamma)$, where γ is the prior probability of exceeding δ, then:

$$\sigma_0^2 = 4[z(1 - \alpha) + z(1 - \beta)]^2 \times \sigma_0^2/[N \cdot z(1 - \gamma)^2] \qquad (9.12)$$

Combining these equations and substituting $2\sigma/N_0$ for σ_0, gives:

$$N_0/N = z(1 - \gamma)^2/[z(1 - \alpha) + z(1 - \beta)]^2 \qquad (9.13)$$

where N_0/N is the 'handicap' of the previous section.

To illustrate the use of the enthusiast and sceptical priors, we consider a hypothetical trial with failure events as the response endpoint. A new and a standard treatment are to be compared by means of the logarithm of the hazard ratio, with the enthusiasts expecting to see a hazard ratio of 2 in favour of the new treatment. The enthusiasts' prior is assumed normal and is centred on $\ln(2) = 0.693$. The sceptics' prior is normal and centred on zero (corresponding to an expected hazard ratio of 1). With common variance equal to $(0.693/1.645)^2$ or 0.176, the sceptics expect an effect size as large as the enthusiasts' mean only 5% of the time. The sceptics' prior can be considered as corresponding to a hypothetical dataset in which the hazard ratio is 1 and there have been 22.7 failures $((n_1 + n_2) = 4/0.176)$.

At an interim analysis, there are 30 events under the old treatment and 10 under the new, with an estimated hazard ratio of 2.9. These data can be represented by a normal distribution centred on $\log(2.9) = 1.065$, with variance $(1/30) + (1/10) = 0.133$.

The enthusiasts are jubilant. Under their prior, the posterior is centred on $\mu_p = (0.693 \times 22.7 + 1.065 \times 40)/(22.7 + 40) = 0.930$ with variance $4/(22.7 + 40) = 0.064$ (standard deviation 0.252). For the enthusiasts, the probability of the hazard ratio being greater than, say, 1.5 is $1 - \phi((\log(1.5) - 0.930)/0.252) = 1 - 0.019 = 0.981$. They would be happy for the trial to be stopped early.

However, combing these data with the prior of the sceptics gives a posterior distribution, with mean $\mu_p = (0 \times 22.7 + 1.065 \times 40)/(22.7 + 40) = 0.679$ and variance $4/(22.7 + 40) = 0.064$. This posterior distribution assigns probability $1 - \phi((0.405 - 0.679)/0.252) = 1 - 0.139 = 0.861$ to the hazard ratio, being greater than 1.5. This might not be sufficient to persuade the sceptic that the trial should be stopped.

9.9. SAMPLE SIZE ESTIMATION FOR EARLY PHASE TRIALS

The previous section has described Bayesian inferential procedures that could be used in the design and analysis of a phase III trial. However, in the early, more exploratory stages of the development of a new therapy, the case for a Bayesian decision theory approach is stronger. The application of decision theory requires the specification of a *gain function*. In some circumstances, the gain function may be concerned with maximising the relevant information gathered from a particular experiment. In others it may express on a common scale the various costs of an experiment and the possible patient suffering or benefit from the experiment. We briefly consider each of these.

Whitehead and Brunier (1995) consider the context of a phase-I dose-finding experiment. Patients are treated one-at-a-time and the response of each patient is observed before the next is treated. They consider a model in which the probability that the ith patient given a dose d_i suffers an adverse reaction follows a logit model of the form:

$$\log \frac{p_i(\theta)}{(1 - p_i(\theta))} = \log \theta_1 + \theta_2 \log(d_i) \tag{9.14}$$

and a generalisation of the simple conjugate beta distribution (see Section 9.2) for the prior distribution for θ is chosen. The objective of the experiment is specified as finding the dose D^* at which an acceptable probability p of adverse reaction is obtained. For example, for $p = 0.2$, then:

$$\log(0.2/0.8) = \log \theta_1 + \theta_2 \log D^* \tag{9.15}$$

In order to minimise the variance in the estimate of D^*, the gain function is specified so as to obtain $G(\theta, d) = \text{Var}(\hat{D}(d)^*)^{-1}$. The design action A_i that will maximise the expected gain, given the information available from the first i patients, is given by:

$$\int G(\theta, d) h(\theta | y_i) d\theta \tag{9.16}$$

where $h(\theta | y_i)$ is the posterior density of θ given the observed responses up to subject i. In general, numerical methods are required to solve for A_i, the optimal next dose.

Although the choice of dose is data dependent, tending to fall if previous responses are adverse or rise if not, maximum-likelihood estimation of dose-response models to the resulting data remains unaffected.

Now consider a phase-II trial. The decision to undertake a phase II trial should take into account possible subsequent gain and loss. Brunier and Whitehead (1994) consider the possible gains laid out in Table 9.3.

In deciding to continue to the phase III trial, they argue that it is intuitively reasonable to continue if a critical number c of the n phase II patients are successfully treated. They then propose a gain function parametrised in terms of n and c:

$$G(n, c) = \int_0^1 h_0(p)(p - p_0)\{n + A_n(p, c)(m + B(p)w)\}dp \tag{9.17}$$

Table 9.3. Gain Function for a Phase II Trial.
Gained Successes.

During Phase II	During Phase III	After Phase III
$n(p - p_0)$	$m(p - p_0)$	$w(p - p_0)$

p = true probability of success of new treatment.

p_0 = probability of success on standard treatment.

n = number of patients given new treatment in phase II trial.

m = number of patients given each treatment in a subsequent phase III trial.

w = number of patients receiving the recommended treatment after the phase III trial.

where

$h_0(p)$ = prior for p

$A_n(p, c)$ = is the probability that the new treatment progresses from phase II to phase III

$$= \sum_{S=c+1}^{n} \binom{n}{S} p^S (1-p)^{(n-S)}$$

$B(p)$ = the power function of the phase III trial

Other quantities are defined in Table 9.3.

Summarising the hypothetical results of the phase III trial as successes S and failures F and total marginal totals T, with subscripts N and C for new and control treatments, then $B(p)$ is given by:

$$1 - \Phi\left(\frac{(k - \theta V)}{\sqrt{(V)}}\right) \tag{9.18}$$

where

$$V = T_N T_C S F / T^3$$

$$\theta = \log \frac{(p_N(1 - p_C))}{(p_C(1 - p_N))}$$

and k is the critical normal deviate at the chosen significance level α.

The analysis may be extended to also consider the costs of trials.

As a consequence of varying the design parameters, they conclude that the optimal size of the phase II trial:

- decreases with the precision of the prior $h_0(p)$
- increases with the size of the 'patient horizon' w
- decreases by using a realistic Phase III power function $B(p)$
- decreases with increasing phase II trial cost
- increases (generally) with increasing phase III trial cost.

The use of a decision analysis approach within the context of an equivalence trial is discussed by Lindley (1998), contrasting the conclusions with those reached using standard frequentist methods.

9.10. REPORTING OF RESULTS

Not surprisingly, the Bayesian perspective suggests that the reporting of trial results could, with advantage, take a rather different form to the traditional frequentist one. In conformity with the general trend, Parmar *et al.* (1994) argue against the focus on p-values. They argue that studies should persuade reasonable sceptics and enthusiasts alike. This is particularly important for sequential trials that are now very common. The use of the sceptical prior acts to reduce the risk of premature stopping of a trial in which some benefit is shown early in the trial. The use of the enthusiastic prior is to reduce the risk of premature stopping due to early lack of benefit. In both cases, the amount of 'pull-back' is much greater in the early stages of a trial when there is relatively little data as compared to the information content of the prior. Freedman, Spiegelhalter and Parmar (1994) suggest that results sections should include the usual tables, curves, estimates and standard errors based on the data, and that interpretation sections should describe prior distributions and give treatment difference estimates (point and interval) using unadjusted (uninformative prior), sceptical and enthusiasts prior. For each prior, a table with probabilities of treatment difference falling below, within and above the range of equivalence should be presented.

9.11. SUMMARY

Although still unfamiliar to some statisticians and regulators, the use of Bayesian methods in the design and analysis of clinical trials is becoming increasingly common. We have done little more than sketch some of the key ideas and procedures in Bayesian estimation and analysis. With faster computation and improvements in theory and associated algorithms, virtually all statisticians involved in trials are likely to find themselves using Bayesian technology. To do so often does not require an acceptance of the use of subjective probability. However, progress is being made in formalising procedures that do use subjective probability. When combined with explicit gain functions into a formal decision framework, the approach is clearly well suited to guiding the research strategy of a group of investgators sharing a common interest. However, we are yet to see whether these will gain longer term acceptance in the more public arena of definitive trials. Bayesian methods are now also much used for meta-analysis, the subject of the final chapter.

CHAPTER 10

Meta-Analysis

10.1. INTRODUCTION

In the *Cambridge Dictionary of Statistics in the Medical Sciences*, meta-analysis is defined thus:

A collection of techniques whereby the results of two or more independent studies are statistically combined to yield an overall answer to a question of interest. The rationale behind this approach is to provide a test with more power than is provided by the separate studies themselves. The procedure has become increasingly popular in the last decade or so, but is not without its critics, particularly because of the difficulties of knowing which studies should be included and to which population final results actually apply.

In essence, meta-analysis is a more systematic approach to combining evidence from multiple research projects than the classical review article. Chalmers and Lau (1993) make the point that both approaches can be biased, but that at least the writer of a meta-analytic paper is required by the rudimentary standards of the discipline to give the data on which the conclusions are based, and to defend the development of these conclusions by giving evidence that all available data are included, or to give the reasons for not including the data. In contrast, the typical reviewer arrives at conclusions that may be biased and then selects data to back them up.

Chalmers and Lau conclude, "It seems obvious that a discipline which requires that all available data be revealed and included in an analysis has an advantage over one that has traditionally not presented analyses of all the data on which conclusions are based."

So meta-analysis is likely to have an objectivity that is inevitably lacking in literature reviews and can also achieve greater precision and generalisability of findings than any single study. Consequently, it is not surprising that the technique has become one of the greatest growth areas in medical research. Some examples of its use are given in Chalmers (1987), Louis, Fienberg and Mosteller (1985), and DerSimonian and Laird (1986). There remain, however, sceptics who feel that the conclusions drawn from meta-analysis often go beyond what the techniques and the data justify. Some of their concerns are echoed in the last part of the definition with which this chapter began, and in the following quotation from Oakes (1993);

The term meta-analysis refers to the quantitative combination of data from independent trials. Where the result of such combination is a descriptive summary of the weight of the available evidence, the exercise is of undoubted value. Attempts to apply inferential methods, however, are subject to considerable methodological and logical difficulties. The selection and quality of the trials included, population bias and the specification of the population to which inference may properly be made are problems to which no satisfactory solutions have been proposed.

Despite such concerns, there has been a striking increase in published meta-analyses of clinical trials. Most stem from the fact that so many trials are too small for adequate conclusions to be drawn about potentially small advantages of particular therapies. Advocacy of large trials is a natural response to this situation, but it is not always possible to launch very large trials before therapies become widely accepted or rejected prematurely. In fact, there are now several instances of very large trials being started after meta-analysis of multiple small ones were strongly positive (see Antman *et al.*, 1992). In this way the use of meta-analysis implies that the whole question of power and sample size determination considered in Chapter 2 needs to be re-evaluated. In Freiman *et al.* (1978), investigators about to undertake a randomised controlled trial are recommended to consult a biostatistician for help in estimating the number of patients to obtain a useful answer, and if the answer were more patients than might be available, to abandon the trial. In a later paper, however, one of the authors confesses to a dramatic change of heart and suggests that the second recommendation is one which is very poor. (See Chalmers and Lau, 1993.)

In this chapter, we shall give a number of examples of meta-analysis and address some of the issues of most concern when applying the method. We begin with perhaps the most important component of any proposed meta-analysis, namely the selection of which studies to include.

10.2.   SELECTION OF STUDIES — WHAT TO INCLUDE

The selection of the studies to be integrated by a meta-analysis will clearly have a bearing on the conclusions reached. Selection is a matter of inclusion and exclusion and the judgements required are often difficult: should only randomised trials be included; should poor quality research be excluded (and who should judge quality?); should only a single endpoint be analysed? — and so on. A great deal of attention has been paid to those issues and there is no consensus view. Chalmers and Lau (1993), aware of the many opportunities to change the results of a meta-analysis by selecting trials the conclusions of which agree with preconceived notions and reject those that do not, suggest the rather involved process outlined in Fig. 10.1 for minimising bias. Blinding papers by blotting out the sources and disguising the results allows 'quality' to be scored in an unbalanced fashion.

Pocock (1993) suggests that the process of selection has three components: breadth, quality and representativeness. Breadth relates to the decision as to whether to study a very specific narrow

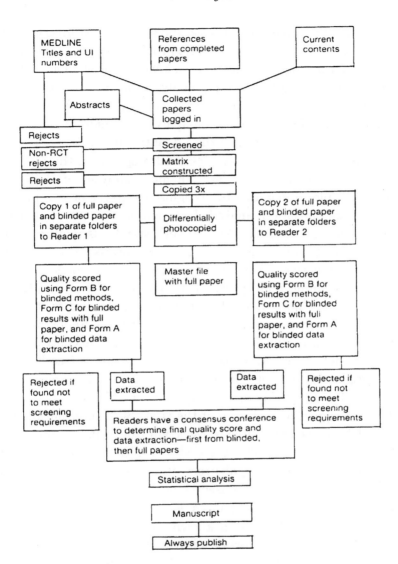

Fig. 10.1. A possible approach for minimising bias when selecting studies to include in a meta-analysis (taken with permission from Chalmers and Lau, 1993).

question (e.g., the same drug, disease and setting for studies following a common protocol) or a more generic problem (e.g., a broad class of treatments for a range of conditions in a variety of settings). Pocock suggests that the broader the meta-analysis, the more difficulty there is in interpreting the combined evidence as regards future policy; consequently, the broader the meta-analysis the more it needs to be interpreted qualitatively rather than quantitatively.

The reliability of a meta-analysis will depend on the quality of the data in the included studies. In meta-analyses of clinical trials, for example, adherence to recognised criteria of acceptability (blinding, randomisation, analysis by intention to treat, etc.) should be looked for, and any relaxation of such standards requires careful consideration as to whether the consequent precision of more data is counter-productive, given the increased potential for loss of credibility. Determining quality would be helped if the results from so many trials were not so poorly reported. In the future, this may be improved by the Consolidation of Standards for Reporting Trials (CONSORT) statement (Begg *et al.*, 1996). The core contribution of the CONSORT statement consists of a flow diagram (see Fig. 10.2) and a checklist (see Table 10.1). The flow diagram enables reviewers and readers to quickly grasp how many eligible participants were randomly assigned to each arm of the trial. Such information is frequently difficult or impossible to ascertain from trial reports as they are currently presented. The checklist identifies 21 items that should be incorporated in the title, abstract, introduction, methods, results or conclusion of every randomised clinical trial.

Ensuring that a meta-analysis is truly representative can be problematic. It has long been known that journal articles are not a representative sample of work addressed to any particular area of research (see, for example, Sterlin, 1959, Greenwald, 1975 and Smith, 1980). Significant research findings, in particular, are more likely to find their way into journals than non-significant results. An informal method of assessing the effect of publication bias is the so-called *funnel plot*, in which effect size from a study is plotted against the

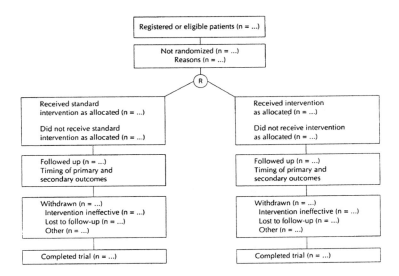

Fig. 10.2. Flow diagram of CONSORT statement.

Table 10.1. Checklist for the CONSORT Statement.

Head. Subhead.	Descriptor	Was it reported?	On what page number?
Title	Identify the study as a randomised trial.		
Abstract	Use a structured format.		
Meth. Protocol	Describe Planned study population, together with inclusion/ exclusion criteria.		
	Planned interventions and their timing.		
	Primary and secondary outcome measure(s) and the minimum important difference(s) and indicate		

Table 10.1. (*Continued*)

Head. Subhead.	Descriptor	Was it reported?	On what page number?
	indicate how the target sample size was projected.		
	Rationale and methods for statistical analyses, detailing main comparative analyses and whether they were completed on an intention-to-treat basis.		
	Prospectively defined stopping rules (if warranted).		
Assignment	Describe unit of randomisation (e.g., individual, cluster, geographic).		
	Method used to generate the allocation schedule.		
	Method of allocation, concealment and timing of assignment.		
	Method to separate the generator from the executor of assigment.		
Masking (Blinding)	Describe mechanism (e.g., capsules, tablets); similarity of treatment characteristics (e.g., appearance, taste) allocation schedule control (location of code during		

Table 10.1 (*Continued*)

Head. Subhead.	Descriptor	Was it reported?	On what page number?
	trial and when broken); and evidence for successful blinding among participants, person doing intervention outcome assessors and data analysts.		
Results: Participant flow and follow-up	Provide a trial profile (figure) summarising participant flow, numbers and timing of randomisation assign-ment, interventions and measurements for each randomised group.		
Analysis	State estimated effect of intervention on primary and secondary outcome measures, including a point estimate and measure of precision (confidence interval).		
	State results in absolute numbers where feasible (e.g., 10/20, not 50%).		
	Present summary data and appropriate descriptive and inferential statistics in sufficient detail to allow for alternative analyses and replication.		

Table 10.1 (*Continued*)

Head. Subhead.	Descriptor	Was it reported?	On what page number?
	Describe prognostic variables by treatment group and any attempt tp adjust for them.		
	Describe protocol deviations form the study as planned, together with the reasons.		
Comment	State specific interpretation of study findings, including sources of bias and imprecision (internal validity) and discussion of external validity, including appropriate quantitative measures when possible.		
	State general interpretation of the data in light of the totality of the available evidence.		

study's sample size. Because of the nature of sampling variability, this plot should, in the absence of publication bias, have the shape of a pyramid with a tapering 'funnel-like' peak. Publication bias will tend to skew the pyramid by selectively excluding studies with small, non-significant effects. Such studies predominate when the sample sizes are small, but are likely to be increasingly less common as the sample sizes increase. Consequently, their absence removes part of the left hand corner of the pyramid. The effect is illustrated in Fig. 10.3.

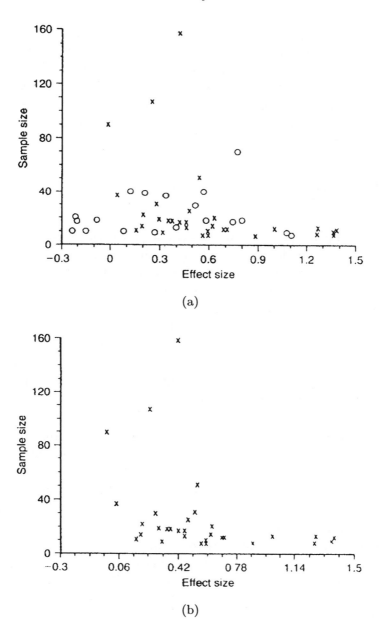

(a)

(b)

Fig. 10.3. Funnel plot.

A meta-analysis that relies solely upon published data is liable to be biased, and confidence in the overall quality of a meta-analysis will be greatly enhanced if explicit efforts are made to identify *all* studies and not just those that are published. This can often be a formidable enterprise possibly taking several years, but there is little doubt that such efforts considerably reduce the danger of overestimating treatment efficacy.

10.3.   THE STATISTICS OF META-ANALYSIS

A meta-analysis should almost always begin with some form of graphical display. A single figure displaying point estimates and confidence intervals for the individual studies is often sufficient to show, at a glance, what the broad conclusions of the analysis are. Figure 10.4, for example, shows the results from a series of randomised controlled trials of endoscopic treatment of bleeding peptic ulcer (see Sacks *et al.*, 1990). The binary outcome variable in each case was whether or not there was a reduction in recurrent or continued bleeding. The results are presented as confidence intervals for the odds ratios. Although four of the 25 trials favour the control group, the overall effect of endoscopic therapy appears to be highly statistically significant.

For some meta-analyses, a diagram such as Fig. 10.4 might be so clear that more detailed statistical investigation becomes unnecessary. In some circumstances, however, investigators might be interested in a global test of significance for the overall null hypothesis of no effect in all studies, or, more commonly, an overall estimate of the magnitude of the effect. Concentrating on the latter, suppose that there are N studies to be analysed. There are two distinct approaches to providing an estimate of overall effect size in a meta-analysis. The first (and most commonly used) is to take the N studies as the only ones of interest. The second is to regard the N studies as a sample from a larger population of relevant studies. The two approaches correspond, respectively, to the assumptions

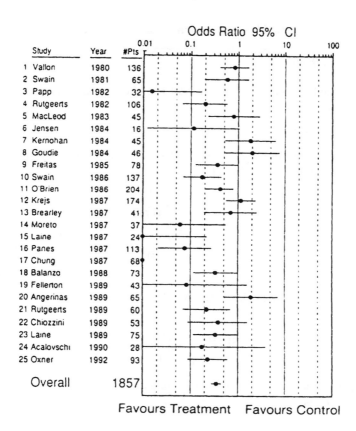

Fig. 10.4. Confidence intervals for odds ratios from a series of randomised trials of endoscopic treatment of bleeding peptic ulcer (from Sacks *et al.*, 1990).

of a fixed and random set of studies for the analysis of variance. Table 10.2 presents the basis of estimation for each approach for a general measure of effect size.

The fixed effect estimate is reliant on the strong assumption that there is no true heterogeneity between studies, i.e., they are all estimating the same true effect and only differ because of sampling variation. Such an assumption can be tested (see Table 10.2), but the

Table 10.2. The Statistical Basis of Meta-Analysis.

(a) *Fixed effects*

- Let Y denote the generic measure of the effect of an experimental intervention (the *effect size*).

- Let W denote the reciprocal of the variance of effect size.

- Under the assumption of a fixed set of studies, an estimator of the assumed common underlying effect size is:

$$\bar{Y} = \frac{\sum\limits_{i=1}^{N} W_i Y_i}{\sum\limits_{i=1}^{N} W_i}$$

- The standard error of this estimator is:

$$\text{SE}(\bar{Y}) = \left[\sum_{i=1}^{N} W_i \right]^{-1/2}$$

- An approximate $100(1-\alpha)\%$ confidence interval for the population effect size, say ψ, is:

$$\bar{Y} - z_{\alpha/2} \Big/ \sqrt{\sum_{i=1}^{N} W_i} \leq \psi \leq \bar{Y} + z_{\alpha/2} \Big/ \sqrt{\sum_{i=1}^{N} W_i}$$

(b) *Random effects*

- Under the assumption that the studies are a random sample from a larger population of studies, there is a mean population effect size, say $\bar{\psi}$, about which the study-specific effect sizes vary. Thus, even if each study's results were based on sample sizes so large that the standard errors of the Ys were zero, there would still be study-to-study variation because each study would have its own underlying effect size (i.e., its own parameter value).

Table 10.2. (*Continued*)

- Let D denote the variance of the studies' effect sizes (a quantity yet to be determined) and let Q denote the following statistic for measuring study-to-study variation in effect size:

$$Q = \sum_{i=1}^{N} W_i (Y_i - \bar{Y})^2 .$$

- The estimated component of variance due to interstudy variation in effect size, D, is calculated as:

$$D = 0 \quad \text{if } Q \leq N - 1$$

$$D = [Q - (N - 1)]/U \quad \text{if } Q > N - 1$$

(see Der Simonian and Laird, 1986) where

$$U = (N - 1)\left[\bar{W} - \frac{S_W^2}{N\bar{W}}\right]$$

with $\bar{W}$ and S_W^2 being the mean and variance of the Ws.

- An approximate $100(1 - \alpha)\%$ confidence interval for $\bar{\psi}$ is:

$$\bar{Y}^* - z_{\alpha/2}/\sqrt{\sum_{i=1}^{N} W_i^*} \leq \bar{\psi} \leq \bar{Y}^* + z_{\alpha/2}/\sqrt{\sum_{i=1}^{N} W_i^*} .$$

where

$$W_i^* = (D + W_i^{-1})^{-1}$$

$$\bar{Y}^* = \frac{\displaystyle\sum_{i=1}^{N} W_i^* Y_i}{\displaystyle\sum_{i=1}^{N} W_i^*}$$

Table 10.2. (*Continued*)

- The confidence interval for the underlying parameter is wider in the random effects model than in the fixed effects model. A random effects analysis suggest more uncertainty in estimating the underlying parameter than does a fixed effects analysis.

- Test for homogeneity of studies — the test statistic; Q is given by:

$$Q = \sum_{i=1}^{N} W_i (Y_i - \bar{Y})^2$$

- The hypothesis of a common effect size is rejected if Q exceeds χ^2_{N-1} at the chosen significance level.

---

test lacks power. Consequently, when such a test is non-significant we cannot assert that the fixed effect method is correct but only that *major* heterogeneity is not present. But in most applications of meta-analysis, homogeneity is *a priori* implausible given the variety of study designs.

The random effects method attempts to incorporate statistical heterogeneity into the overall estimate of an average effect. According to Fleiss (1993) "the random effects model anticipates better than the fixed effects model the possibility that some studies not included in the analysis are underway, are about to be published, or perhaps have even already been published in a obscure journal, and that the results in some of the non-included studies are different from the results in most of the meta-analysed studies". Again in a report on combining information sponsored by the National Research Council's Committee on Applied and Theoretical Statistics (National Research Council, 1992) the conclusion is that "modeling would be improved by an increase in the use of random effects models in preference to the current default of fixed effects models."

But Pocock (1993) suggests that the random effects method has both conceptual and practical problems; he dislikes both the assumptions that the studies are a random sample from a hypothetical population of such studies, and that if heterogeneity exists, that substantially more weight is given to the smaller studies than in the fixed effect approach when smaller studies are often those of poorer quality. The problem is usually not too serious provided that the number of patients in a given trial is not too small — the problem becomes less not as the number of trials increases but as the number of patients per trial increases.

Thompson (1993) also raises some doubts about the random effects model, arguing that it may mask the true reasons for the underlying heterogeniety and that possible explanations should be investigated. One possibility would be to use generalised linear models (see Chapters 4 and 7) allowing for both fixed study level covariates, indicating characteristics of the study that may be related to effect size and thought to explain some of the heterogeneity, together with a random component to accomodate unexplained heterogeneity.

DeMets (1987) and Bailey (1987) discuss the strengths and weaknesses of the two competing models. Bailey, for example, suggests that when the research question involves extrapolation into the future — *Will* the treatment have an effect, on the average? — then the random effects model for the studies is the appropriate one. This research question implicitly assumes that there is a population of studies from which those analysed in the meta-analysis were sampled, and anticipates future studies being conducted or previously unknown studies being uncovered. In contrast, when the research questions concern whether treatment *has* produced an effect, on the average *in the set of studies being analysed*, then the fixed effects model is the one-to-use. Meier (1987) and Peto (1987) present further arguments in favour of one or other of the models.

Oakes (1993) also considers the methodological arguments that can arise in the application of meta-analysis, but in addition, addresses the wider question of whether the statistical combination of results from different trials is legitimate at all. He makes the point that the principal feature of statistical inference is the argument from sample to population. For the argument to have pretensions to strict legitimacy, the sample must be the result of a random process; for the argument to make sense, the population must be identifiable. In the case of meta-analysis, Oakes argues that there are grounds for concern on both counts, and at the heart of the debate as to whether and to what extent data from differing studies may legitimately be combined — the so-called problem of apples and oranges — is the question of "what is the population?" Without a clear conception of the population, Oakes suggests that a parameter or its meta-analytic estimate is meaningless, and devoid of application. Oakes finally summarises his own views about applying the inferential process in meta-analysis as follows:

It is my guess that the controversial inferential aspect of meta-analysis, like the positivist philosophy to which it is the witting or unwitting heir, will not fall to sceptical critiques such as mine but rather it will collapse under its own weight in the conscientious application of its practitioners.

Researchers will move effortlessly from the insightful collection, stratification and summary of disparate results to the intelligent interpretation of them. The specious pseudo-objective accuracy of the intervening statistical inferences will be discreetly dropped.

Medical science will not suffer.

Table 10.3. Results from Nine Trials Comparing SMFP and NaF Toothpastes in Prevention of Caries Development.

Study	NaF			SMFP			SMFP-NaF
	n	Mean	SD	n	Mean	SD	
1	134	5.96	4.24	113	4.72	4.72	+0.86
2	175	4.74	4.64	151	5.07	5.38	+0.33
3	137	2.04	2.59	140	2.51	3.22	+0.47
4	184	2.70	2.32	179	3.20	2.46	+0.50
5	174	6.09	4.86	169	5.81	5.14	−0.28
6	754	4.72	5.33	736	4.76	5.29	0.04
7	209	101.0	8.10	209	10.90	7.90	+0.80
8	1151	2.82	3.05	1122	3.01	3.32	+0.019
9	679	3.88	4.85	673	4.37	5.37	+0.49

Like Thompson and Pocock (1991), it appears that Oakes views meta-analysis as largely an objective descriptive technique and plays down the value of the quantitative results of such an analysis. But the growing use of meta-analysis in a number of speciality areas with quantitative results being regarded at least as importantly as those that are qualitative, argues that in practice meta-analysis is seen as more substantial than a mere descriptive technique.

10.4. TWO EXAMPLES OF THE APPLICATION OF META-ANALYSIS

10.4.1. The Comparison of Sodium Monofluorophosphate (SMFP) and Sodium Fluoride (NaF) Toothpastes in the Prevention of Caries Development

Table 10.3 shows the results of nine randomised trials comparing SMFP and NaF toothpastes for the prevention of caries development. The outcome in each trial was the change, from baseline, in the decayed, missing (due to caries) and filled surface (DMFS) dental index. Calculation of the test for heterogeneity given in Table 10.2 leads to a value for Q of 5.40. Testing this as a chi-squared with 8 degrees of freedom provides no evidence of heterogeniety in the nine trials; consequently, only the fixed effects model will be used. Applying the general methodology described in Table 10.2 to the mean differences leads to a pooled estimate of the effect size of 0.283 with a 95% confidence interval of $(0.103, 0.464)$. The trials provide convincing evidence of a greater change from baseline in the DMFS index when using toothpastes containing SMFP than when using pastes containing NaF.

10.4.2. The Effectiveness of Aspirin in Preventing Death after a Myocardial Infarction

Table 10.4 shows the results of seven randomised trials, in chronological order, of the effectiveness of aspirin (versus placebo) in preventing

Table 10.4. Results of Seven Trials of Aspirin for Preventing Death after a Myocardial Infarction.

		Survived	Died	Total
1. Elwood *et al.*	Aspirin	566	49	615
(1974)	Placebo	557	67	624
	Total	1123	116	1239
2. Coronary drug	Aspirin	714	44	758
project group (1976)	Placebo	707	64	77
	Total	1421	108	1529
3. Elwood and	Aspirin	730	102	832
Sweetnam (1979)	Placebo	724	126	850
	Total	1454	228	1682
4. Breddin *et al.*	Aspirin	285	32	317
(1979)	Placebo	271	38	309
	Total	556	70	626
5. Persantine-Aspirin	Aspirin	725	85	810
Study Group (1980)	Placebo	354	52	406
	Total	1079	137	1216
6. Aspirin study	Aspirin	2021	346	2267
Group (1980)	Placebo	2038	219	2257
	Total	4059	465	4524
7. ISIS-2 Collaborative	Aspirin	7017	1570	8587
Group (1988)	Placebo	6880	1720	8600
	Total	13897	3290	17187

death after a myocardial infarction (the data are taken from Fleiss, 1993). In this case, a suitable measure of effect size is the logarithm of the odds ratio (see Chapter 4). The meta-analysis results are given in Table 10.5. The fixed effects model indicates a positive effect for aspirin, but using the random effects approach, the confidence interval for the overall odds ratio expands to include the value one, indicating no effect.

Table 10.5. A Meta-analysis of the Data in Table 10.4.

(a) *Fixed effects*

Study	Odds Ratio	log(odds ratio)	$W = 1/\text{VAR}[\log(or)]$
1	1.18	0.17	24.09
1	1.47	0.38	24.29
3	1.25	0.22	48.80
4	1.25	0.22	15.44
5	1.25	0.23	27.41
6	0.88	−0.12	103.99
7	1.12	0.11	663.92

Using log(or) as the measure of effect size we have:

$$\bar{Y} = 0.104$$

and a 95% confidence interval for the logarithm of the population odds ratio is $(0.039, 0.169)$.

With respect to the odds ratio itself, the point estimate is 1.109 and the confidence interval is $(1.040, 1.184)$.

(b) *Random effects*

Again using log(or) as the measure of effect size, the various quantities defined in Table 10.1 are as follows:

$$\bar{W} = 129.85$$

$$S_W^2 = 56363.38$$

$$U = 345.02$$

$$D = 0.008$$

$$Q = 8.76$$

$$\bar{Y}^* = 0.1158$$

$$W_1^* \cdots W_7^* = 20.19, 20.33, 35.09, 17.74, 23.14, 56.74, 105.11$$

The 95% confidence for the logarithm of the population odds ratio is $(-0.0025, 0.2341)$.

With respect to the odds ratio itself, the point estimate is 1.123 and the confidence interval is $(0.997, 1.263)$.

10.5. BAYESIAN META-ANALYSIS

A Bayesian approach to meta-analysis might begin with the following random effects model:

$$Y_i \sim N(\theta_i, \sigma_i^2/n_i) \tag{10.1}$$

$$\theta_i \sim N(\bar{\psi}, \tau^2) \quad i = 1, \ldots, N \tag{10.2}$$

where θ_i is the true but unknown effect in the ith study and $\bar{\psi}$ is the unknown population effect; it is the latter quantity which is of most interest, since it represents the pooled effect indicated by the studies. Finally, τ^2 is the population variance, or the between-study variability, and is also of interest since it is a measure of how variable the effect is within a population. In the case where $\tau^2 = 0$, a fixed effect model is obtained.

In a Bayesian setting, prior distributions would be needed for the unknown parameters of the model. A normal prior is typically specified for $\bar{\psi}|\tau$. Although a prior for τ could be specified, for example specifying the precision, $1/\tau$, as being gamma distributed (see Section 9.3 for such a specification for the variance of a random effect for frailty), such a specification is not necessary. With a prior for τ, $\pi(\tau)$, the posterior distribution for τ given the observed effect sizes $f(\tau|Y)$ is proportional to:

$$\pi(\tau) \exp\left(-\sum_{i=1}^{N} \frac{(Y_i - \bar{\psi})}{2 * S_i}\right) \left[\Pi_{i=1}^{N} S_i \times \sum_{i=1}^{N} \frac{1}{S_i}\right]^{-\frac{1}{2}} \tag{10.3}$$

where $S_i = \tau^2 + (\sigma_i^2/n_i)$

Assuming a uniform distribution for $\pi(\tau)$, the posterior distribution can then be approximated by a discrete distribution calculated over, say, 100 equally spaced points that straddle its mode and with a range sufficient to include all the values in which the density is at least 1% of that at the mode (Hedges, 1998). The simple sum of the 100-point densities provides the normalising constant.

With $f(\tau|Y)$ approximated by this discrete distribution, a posterior density for $\bar{\psi}|Y$ is easily calculated as a finite mixture of the conditional densities $g(\bar{\psi}|Y,\tau)$. This conditional density is Normal with mean:

$$\bar{\psi} = \sigma^2(\tau) \sum_{i=1}^{n} \frac{Y_i}{S_i} \tag{10.4}$$

and variance

$$\sigma^2(\tau) = \left(\sum_{i=1}^{n} \frac{1}{S_i} \right)^{-1} \tag{10.5}$$

giving the posterior density for $\bar{\psi}$ as:

$$g(\bar{\psi}|Y) = \int_0^{\infty} \Phi\left(\frac{\tau - \bar{\tau}}{\sigma(\tau)} \right) f(\tau|Y) d\tau \tag{10.6}$$

where $\Phi(x)$ is the standard normal probability density function.

Monte Carlo methods provide an alternative means of calculating $g(\bar{\psi}|Y)$. A value of τ is first sampled from $f(\tau|Y)$, and then a value for $\bar{\psi}$ is drawn from $f(\bar{\psi}|Y,\tau)$.

A plot of the estimated posterior density $g(\bar{\psi}|Y)$ provides a useful graphical expression for the uncertainty in $\bar{\psi}$. A mean and variance can be calculated as, too, can the probability that the mean effect size is positive, or above some other clinically meaningful value.

In principle, the Bayesian approach has the advantage over the methods of the previous section for random effects models, of more completely accounting for the uncertainty in the estimation of the random effect in the standard errors and confidence intervals of the overall effect estimate. In practice, the results calculated using Bayesian methods differ little from those using the methods of the previous sections unless the number of studies is very small or the studies are very variable. It is also under these circumstances that the particular choice of prior for τ may have a substantial impact. It is therefore important to examine the sensitivity of findings to different choices of prior.

Kass and Wasserman (1996) provide some useful background for the choice of prior distributions. For $\tau = 0$, the Bayesian estimates of the study specific effects are all equal to the common fixed effect estimate. When τ is very large in proportion to the within study sampling variance, then the Bayesian estimates approach their observed values. For intermediate values of τ, the estimates lie between their observed values and the overall common mean — they are 'shrunken' towards the mean, the studies with the more uncertain effect sizes (usually the smaller studies) being more shrunken. Therefore priors for τ that are more concentrated on zero will generate greater shrinkage than more diffuse priors.

However, Bayesian methods are relatively simply modified to consider more general random effects specifications, e.g., to examine the implications of using study effect size distributions with heavier tails, such as Student's t or gamma distributions (e.g., Smith *et al.*, 1995). Analyses with an informative prior for the effect size are also a little more complex.

10.6.   META-ANALYSIS IN MORE COMPLEX SETTINGS

The analyses above have assumed that the contributing studies and their corresponding effect sizes Y_i are exchangeable. No study-level covariates have been considered and are conditional on the θ_i and the Y_i being independent. Non-independence may arise through a clustering of contributing trials by centre, by an overlap of patients across trials, or sometimes by the presence of single studies that provide more than one estimate of effect. In the more complex cases, the question arises as to whether a more effective analysis might be achieved by combining data at the level of the individual subject, i.e., data pooling, rather than at the level of the trial. Senn (1998)

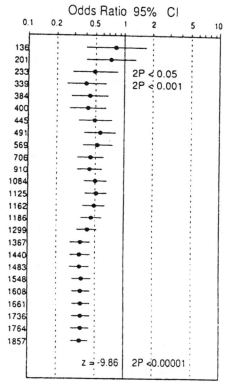

Fig. 10.5. Confidence intervals for odds ratios from a series of randomised trials of endoscopic treatment of bleeding peptic ulcer presented in cumulative form (form Chalmers and Lau, 1993).

considers this question in relation to covariate adjustment, favouring data pooling.

10.7. SUMMARY

Meta-analysis has become one of the greatest growth areas in medical research, despite the many tough criticisms that have been levelled at the approach. (An excellent recent account is available is Normand, 1999.) Users (and potential users) of meta-analysis need to keep in mind the problems that arise at each stage — what studies to select for inclusion; should fixed or random effects models be used to provide an overall estimate of effect size; to what population can results be generalised? And if meta-analysis, despite its wide usage, remains controversial, what can be said of the suggestion of Chalmers and Lau (1993) that *cumulative* meta-analysis might be employed to establish such strong evidence of a treatment effect to make further randomised trials unjustified? Figure 10.5, for example, shows the data previously presented in Fig. 10.4 in a cumulative fashion. Note that by 1982 the chances that endoscopic therapy was not reducing recurrent or continued bleeding, when compared with standard therapy, was less than one in a thousand. Yet in the 25th published trial, patients were randomly assigned to a control group between April 1989 and June 1991. Chalmers and Lau comment, "If the authors of the later publications knew of the previous ones, how much proof did they require, or were they tied to the null hypothesis yoke?" They conclude, "the advent of cumulative meta-analysis makes one worry about the present custom of conducting clinical trials as if no prior trials of the same treatment had been done. When is it no longer ethical to assign patients at random to a control group in a new definitive large trial?"

Software

Many of the methods described in this book could not be applied routinely without the aid of some convenient piece of statistical software. Fortunately, many excellent statistical packages are now widely available, although our intention in this appendix is not to attempt either a comprehensive review or critique. Instead, we shall give details of packages that we feel are most suitable for specific applications and analyses. Links to web pages for a wide variety of statistical software can be found at:

http://www.stata.com/support/links/stat_software.html

1. SOFTWARE FOR SAMPLE SIZE DETERMINATION

nQuery Advisor Version 2.0: A package for choosing an appropriate sample size for many types of design and analysis including two-sample and paired *t*-tests, analysis of variance, crossover designs, nonparametric tests, survival analysis and regression. Very simple to use and well described is the user manual written by Janet D. Elashoff.

Available from:

- Statistical Solutions Ltd. 8 South Bank, Crosse's Green, Cork, Ireland: Tel +353 21 319629, Fax +353 21 319630:

  http://www.statsol.ie:

- In the USA, Boston, MA, USA 1-800-262-1171:

  http://www.statsolusa.com: info@statsolusa.com

MS-DOS 3.1 or higher, Microsoft Windows 3.1, Windows 95 or Windows NT is required.

A large number of other software packages for estimating sample size when designing studies can be found on:

  http://www.interchg.ubc.ca/cacb/power

2. SOFTWARE FOR MULTIPLE IMPUTATION OF MISSING VALUES

Software is available from Statistical Solutions (address above) and from:

  http://www.stat.psu.edu/~jls/misoftwa.html

3. SOFTWARE FOR INTERIM ANALYSIS

- *EaSt, Version 2*: Cytel Software Corporation, 675 Massachusetts Ave., Cambridge, MA 98195, USA.
- *PEST3, Planning and Evaluation of Sequential Trials*: MPS Research Unit, University of Reading, Earley Gate, Reading RG6 6FN, United Kingdom. Both these packages are reviewed in Emerson (1996).

4. SOFTWARE FOR GENERALISED LINEAR MODELS

Generalised linear models can be fitted using most statistical packages, including:

- SAS — SAS Institute Inc., SAS Campus Drive, Cary, NC 27513, USA.

- STATA — Stata Corp., 702, University Drive East, College Station, TX 77840, USA.
- GENSTAT — Numerical Algorithms Group Ltd., Wilkinson House, Jordon Hill Rd., Oxford OX28DR, UK.
- SPSS — SPSS Inc., 444 N. Michigan Ave., Chicago, IL 60611, USA.

5. SOFTWARE FOR ANALYSING LONGITUDINAL DATA

For the summary measure or response feature approach described in Chapter 5, any of the standard packages can be used. For the more involved modelling approaches covered in Chapters 6 and 7 there are a number of possibilities:

5.1 Multivariate normal regression model

Both BMDP5V and SAS PROC MIXED (see, *Getting Started with PROC MIXED*, SAS Institute Inc.) can be used to fit the types of models described in Chapter 6. A variety of structures may be specified for the covariance matrix of the repeated measurements, including independence, compound symmetry, random effects and unstructured.

4.1 Generalized Linear Mixed Models (GLMM)

Three general approaches to GLMM estimation are available.

(1) Maximum likelihood estimation:
- Tractable special cases; binomial mixed logistic in EGRET (Statistics and Epidemiology Research Corp., 1107 NE 45th St., Suite 520, Seattle, WA 98105); negative binomial of Stata's **nbreg**.
- Standard numerical integration; **gllamm** written for STATA. (Computational time can be considerable.)

(2) An approximation based on a linearising adaptation to standard random effects algorithms.

- This is available in SAS (**glimmix**) — downloadable from:

  "http://www.sas.com/techsup/download/samples/ stat_and_iml"

  with documentation by Wolfinger, *Reference for glimmix: a tutorial on mixed models* (SAS Institute Inc.).
- Also available in MLW in — the Multilevel Models Project, Mathematical Sciences, Institute of Education, University of London, 20 Bedford Way, London WC1H0AL, UK.

(3) A Bayesian approach using Monte Carlo Markov Chain estimation. Models may be specified and fitted entirely within an MCMC framework (e.g., BUGS available from **http://www.mrcbsu.cam.ac.uk**) or MCMC may be used as a final stage (e.g., MLWin).

5.2 Generalised Estimating Equations approach

This approach is now available in SAS, STATA and S-PLUS — Statsci Division, MathSoft Inc, 1700 Westlake Avenue N, #500 Seattle, Washington 98109–9891, USA.

5.3 Missing Data

(1) The Diggle/Kenward model for dropouts is implemented in the OSWALD (Object oriented software for the analysis of longitudinal data in S) written by David M. Smith, Bill Robertson and Peter Diggle. The software runs under S or S-Plus on both Unix and DOS systems. OSWALD is available from:

http://www.maths.lancs.ac.uk:2080/∼maa036/oswald/

(2) Weighting approaches for the treatment of missing data can be implemented in SAS, SUDAAN (Research Triangle Institute, P.O. Box 12194, Research Triangle Park, NC 27709, USA), and particularly simply in STATA.

6. SOFTWARE FOR BAYESIAN ANALYSIS

BUGS provides a model specification language allowing a wide variety of models to be estimated via Gibbs sampling. The documentation provides an extensive range of examples.

7. SOFTWARE FOR SURVIVAL ANALYSIS

(1) The routine methods of analysis, such as Kaplan-Meier, Cox's regression, etc., are available in all standard packages such as SAS and SPSS.

(2) A wider range of techniques are implemented in S-Plus and STATA.

(3) A number of other very useful methods are described in *Extending the Cox Model*, Technical Report Number 58, Mayo Clinic, Rochester, Minnesota, written by Professor Terry Therneau.

REFERENCES

Adkinson, N.F., Eggleston, P.A., Eney, D., Goldstein, E.O., Schuberth, K.C., Bacon, J.R., Hamilton, R.G., Weiss, M.E., Arshand, H., Meinert, C.L., Tonascra, J. and Wheeler, B. (1997). A controlled trial of immunotherapy for asthma in allergic children, *New Engl. J. Med.* **336**: 324–331.

Altman, D.G. and De Stavola, B.L. (1994). Practical problems in fitting a proportional hazards model to data with updated measurements of the covariates, *Statist. Med.* **13**: 301–341.

Amberson, J.B., McMahon, B.T. and Pinner, M. (1931). A clinical trial of sanocrysin in pulmonary tuberculosis, *Am. Rev. Tubercul.* **24**: 401–435.

Andersen, B. (1990). *Methodological Errors in Medical Research*, Blackwell Scientific Publications, Oxford.

Anderson, P.K., Borgan, O., Gill, R.D. and Keiding, N. (1993). *Statistical Models Based on Counting Processes*, Springer-Verlag, NY.

Anderson, P.K. and Gill, R.D. (1982). Cox's regression model for counting process: a large sample study, *Ann. Statist.* **10**: 1100–1120.

Anscombe, F.J. (1954). Fixed-sample size analysis of sequential observations, *Biometrics* **10**: 89–100.

Antman, E.M., Lau, J., Jimenez-Silva, J., Kupelnick, B., Mosteller, F. and Chalmers, T.C. (1992). A comparison of results of meta-analysis of randomized control trials and recommendations of clinical experts; treatments for myocardial infarction, *J. Am. Med. Assoc.* **268**: 240–248.

Armitage, P., McPherson, C.K. and Rowe, B.C. (1969). Repeated significance tests on accumulating data, *J. Roy. Statist. Soc. Ser. A* **132**: 235–244.

Armitage, P. (1983). Trials and errors: the emergence of clinical statistics, *J. Roy. Statist. Soc. Ser. A* **146**: 321–334.

Aspirin Myocardia Infarction Study Research Group (1980). A randomised controlled trial of aspirin in persons recovered from myocardial infarction. *J. Am. Med. Assoc.* **243**: 661–669.

Azzalini, A. and Cox, D.R. (1984). Two new tests associated with analysis of variance, *J. Roy. Statist. Soc. Ser. B.*, pp. 335–343.

Bailey, K.R. (1987). Inter-study differences: How should they influence the interpretation and analysis of results? *Statist. in Med.* **6**: 351–358.

Barlow, W.E. and Prentice, R.L. (1988). Residuals for relative risk regressions. *Biometrika* **75**: 65–74.

Beecham, J. and Knapp, M.R.J. (1992). Costing psychiatric interventions. In *Measuring Mental Health Needs* (eds. G. Thornicroft, C. Brewin and J. Wing), Gaskell, London, pp. 163–183.

Begg, C., Cho, M., Eastwood, S., Morton, R., Moher, D., Ohlein, I., *et al.* (1996). Improving the quality of reporting of randomised controlled trials; the CONSORT statement, *J. Am. Med. Assoc.* **276**: 637–939.

Berkey, C.S., Anderson, J.J. and Hoaglen, D.C. (1996). Multiple-outcome meta analysis of clinical trials, *Statist. Med.* **15**: 537–557.

Berry, D.A. (1990). Basic principles in designing and analyzing clinical studies. In *Statistical Methodology in the Pharmaceutical Sciences* (ed. D.A. Berry), Marcel Dekker, New York, pp. 1–55.

Berry, D.A. (1993). A case for Bayesianism in clinical trials, *Statist. Med.* **12**: 1377–1393.

Berzuni, C. (1996). Medical monitoring. In *Markov Chain Monte Carlo in Practice* (eds. W.R. Gilks, S. Richardson and D.J. Spiegelhalter), Chapman and Hall, London, pp. 321–338.

Binder, D.A. (1983). On the variances of asymptotically normal estimators from complex surveys, *Int. Statist. Rev.* **51**: 279–292.

Blair, R.C., Troendle, J.F. and Beck, R.W. (1996). Control of familywise errors in multiple endpoint assessments via stepwise permutation tests, *Statist. Med.* **15**: 1107–1121.

Bracken, M.B. (1987). Clinical trials and the acceptance of uncertainty, *Br. Med. J.* **294**: 111–112.

Bradford Hill, A. (1962). *Statistical Methods in Clinical and Preventative Medicine*, Livingstone, Edinburgh.

Breddin, K., Loew, D., Lechner, K. and Uberla, E.W. (1979). Secondary prevention of myocardial infarction. Comparison of acetylsalicykic acid, phenprcoumon and placebo. A multicenter, two-year prospective study. *Thrombosis and Haemostasis* **41**: 225–236.

Breslow, N.E. (1974). Covariance analysis of censored survival data, *Biometrics* **30**: 89–99.

Breslow, N.E. (1990). Tests of hypotheses in overdispersion regression and other quasi-likelihood models, *J. Am. Statist. Assoc.* **85**: 565–571.

Bruner, H.C. and Whitehead, J. (1994). Sample sizes for phase III clinical trials derived from Bayesian Decision Theory, *Statist. Med.*, 2493-2502.

Byar, D.P. (1985). Assessing apparent treatment — covariate interactions in randomized clinical trials, *Statist. Med.* **4**: 255–263.

Cain, K.C. and Lange, N.T. (1984) Approximate case influence for the proportional hazards regression model with censored data, *Biometrics* **40**: 493–499.

Carey, V., Zeger, S.L. and Diggle, P. (1993). Modelling multivariate binary data with alternating logistic regressions, *Biometrika* **80**: 517–526.

Chalmers, T.C. (1987). Meta-analysis in clinical medicine, *Trans. Am. Clin. Climatol. Assoc.* **99**: 144–150.

Chalmers, T.C. and Lau, J. (1993). Meta-analysis stimulus for change in clinical trials, *Statist. Meth. Med. Res.* **2**: 161–172.

Chalmers, T.C., Matta, R.J., Smith, H. and Kunzler, A.M. (1977). Evidence favouring the use of anticoagulents in the hospital phase of acute myocardial infarction, *N. Engl. J. Med.* **297**: 1091–1096.

Chastang, C., Byar, D. and Piantadosi, S. (1988). A quantitative study of the bias in estimating the treatment effect caused by omitting a balanced covariate in survival models, *Statist. Med.* **7**: 1243–1255.

Chen, C.-H. and Wang, P.C. (1991). Diagnostic plots in Cox's regression model, *Biometrics* **47**: 841–850.

Chesher, A. and Jewitt, I. (1987). The bias of a heteroskedasticity consistent covariance matrix estimator, *Econometrica* **55**: 1217–1222.

Chesher, A and Lancaster, T. (1983) The estimation of models of labour behaviour, *Rev. Econ. Stud.* **50**: 609–624.

Chuang-Stein, C. (1993). The regression fallacy, *Drug Info. J.* **27**: 1213–1220.

Chuang-Stein, C. and Tong, D.M. (1997). The impact and implication of regression to the mean on the design and analysis of medical investigations, *Statist. Meth. Med. Res.* **6**: 115–128.

Clayton, D.G. (1974). Some odds ratio statistics for the analysis of ordered categorical data, *Biometrika* **61**: 525–531.

Cnaan, A., Laird, N.M. and Shasor, P. (1997). Using the general linear mixed model to analyse unbalanced repeated measures and longitudinal data, *Statist. Med.* **16**: 2349–2380.

Collett, D. (1991). *Modelling Binary Data*, Chapman and Hall, London.

Collett, D. (1994). *Modelling Survival Data in Medical Research*, Chapman and Hall, London.

Collins, R. (1993). Capopril, nitrates and magnesium after myocardial infraction: Inetroduction and results — ISIS-4. Quoted from taped presentation. American Heart Association's 66th Scientific sessions, Atlanta, 8–11 November.

Coronary Drug Project Research Group. (1973). The Coronary Drug Project: Design, methods and baseline results. 47 (supplement I), I-1-I-50.

Coronary Drug Project Research Group. (1976). Asprin in coronary heart disease, *J. Chronic Diseases*, **29**: 625–642.

Cornfield, J. (1976). Recent methodological contributions to clinical trials, *Am. J. Epidemiol.* **104**: 408–421.

Cox, D.R. (1972). Regression models and life tables, *J. Roy. Statist. Soc. Ser.* **B34**: 187–220.

Cox, D.R. (1975). Partial likelihood, *Biometrika* **62**: 269–276.

Cox, D.R. (1998). Discussion, *Statist. Med.* **17**: 387-389.

Cox, D.R. and Oakes, D. (1984). *Analysis of Survival Data*, Chapman and Hall, London.

Cox, D.R. and Snell, E.J. (1968). A general definition of residuals. *J. Roy. Statist. Soc. Ser.* **B30**: 248–275.

Cramer, J.A., Collins, J.F. and Mallson, R.H. (1988). Can categorization of patient background problems be used to determine early termination in a clinical trial? *Contr. Clin. Trials* **9**: 47–63.

Crombie, A.C., (1952). Avicenna's influence on the medieval scientific tradition. In *Avicenna: Scientist and Philosopher* (ed. G.M. Wickens), Luzac and Co. Ltd., London, pp. 84–107.

Crouchley, R. and Pickles, A. (1993). Information matrix tests of specification for univariate and multivariate proportional hazards models, *Biometrics* **49**: 1067–1076.

Crowley, J. and Hu, M. (1977). Covariance analysis of heart transplant survival data. *J. Am. Statist. Assoc.* **78**: 27–36.

Crowley, J. and Storer, B.G. (1983). Comment on a re-analysis of the 'Stanford Heart Transplant Data' by Aitkin, Laird and Francis, *J. Am. Statist. Assoc.* **78**: 277–281.

Curran, W.J. and Shapiro, E.D. (1970). *Law, Medicine and Forensic Science*, 2nd ed., Little, Brown and Co, Boston.

Curran, D., Bacchi, M., Schmitz, S.F.H., Molenberghs, G. and Sylvester (1998). Identifying the types of missingness in quality of life cancer clinical trials, *Statist. Med.* **17**: 739–756.

Davis, C.S. (1991). Semi-parametric and non-parametric methods for the analysis of repeated measurements with applications to clinical trials, *Statist. Med.* **10**: 1959–1980.

De Mets, D.L. (1987). Methods for combining randomized clinical trials: Strengths and limitations, *Statist. Med.* **6**: 341–348.

De Mets, D.L. and Lan, K.K.G. (1994). Interim analysis — the alpha spending function approach, *Statist. Med.* **13**: 1341–1352.

Der Simonian, R. and Laird, N. (1986). Meta-analysis in clinical trials, *Contr. Clin. Trials* **7**: 177–186.

Diggle, P.J. (1992). Discussion of Liang, K.-Y., Zeger, S.L. and Qaqish, B. (1992). Multivariate regression analyses for categorical data (with discussion), *J. Roy. Statist. Soc.* **B54**: 3–40.

Diggle, P.J. (1988). An approach to the analysis of repeated measures, *Biometrics* **44**: 959–971.

Diggle, P.J. (1998). Dealing with missing values in longitudinal studies. In *Statistical Analysis of Medical Data: New Developments* (eds. B.S. Everitt and G. Dunn), Arnold, London, pp. 203–228.

Diggle, P.J. and Kenward, M.G. (1994). Informative drop-out in longitudinal analysis (with discussion), *Appl. Statist.* **43**: 49–93.

Diggle, P.J., Liang, K.Y. and Zeger, S.L. (1994). *Analysis of Longitudinal Data*, Oxford Scientific Publications, Oxford.

Donner, A. (1984). Approaches to sample size estimation in the designing of clinical trials — a review, *Statist. Med.* **3**: 199–214.

Donner, A. and Klar, N. (1994). Cluster randomization trials in epidemiology — theory and application, *J. Statist. Plan. Infer.* **42**: 37–56.

Drum, M. and McCullagh, P. (1993). Comment on Fitzmaurice, G.M., Laird, N. and Rotnitzky, A. Regression models for discrete longitudinal responses, *Statist. Sci.* **8**: 284–309.

DuMouchel, W.H. (1990). Bayesian meta-analysis. In *Statistical Methodology in Pharmaceutical Sciences* (ed. D.A. Berry), Marcel Dekker, New York, pp. 509-29.

Dunn, G. (1989). *Design and Analysis of Reliability Studies: Statistical Evaluation of Measurement Errors*, Arnold. London.

Dunn, G. (1999). Compliance in clinical trials, *Statist. Med.*, in press.

Dunn, G., Everitt, B.S. and Pickles, A. (1993). *Modelling Covariances and Latent Variables using EQS*, Chapman and Hall, London.

Efron, B. (1979). Bootstrap methods: another look at the jackknife, *Ann. Statist.* **7**: 1–26.

Efron, B. (1998). Foreword in special issue on Analyzing Non-Compliance in Clinical Trials, *Statist. Medi.* **17**: 249–250

Efron, B. and Feldman, D. (1991). Compliance as an explanatory variable in clinical trials, *J. Am. Statist. Assoc.* **86**: 9–17.

Efron, B. and Tibshirani, R. (1986). Bootstrap measures for standard errors, confidence intervals and other measures of statistical accuracy, *Statist. Sci.* **1**: 54–77.

Elwood, P.C., Cochrane, A.L., Burr, M.L., Sweetnam, P.M., Williams, G., Welsby, E., Hugher, S.J. and Renton, R. (1974). A randomized controlled trial of acetyl solicyclic acid in its secondary prevention of mortality from myocardial infarction, *Brit. Med. J.*, **1**: 436–440.

Elwood, P.C. and Sweetnam, P. (1979). Aspirin and secondary mortality after myocardial infarction, *Lancet* **2**: 1313–1315.

Emerson, S.S. (1996). Statistical packages for group sequential methods, *The Am. Statist.* **50**: 183–192.

Everitt, B.S. (1996). An introduction to finite mixture distributions, *Statist. Meth. Med. Res.* **5**: 107–127.

Fairclough, D.L., Peterson, H.F. and Chang, V. (1998). Why are missing quality of life data a problem in clinical trials of cancer therapy? *Statist. Med.* **17**: 667–678.

Falissard, B. and Lellouch, J. (1992). A new procedure for group sequential analysis in clinical trials, *Biometrics* **48**: 373–388.

Farewell, V.T. (1982). The use of mixture models for the analysis of survival data with longterm survivors. *Biometrics* **38**: 1041–46.

Farewell, V., Fleming, T.R. and Harrington, D.P. (1991). *Counting Processes and Survival Analysis*, John Wiley and Sons, New York.

Feinstein, A.R. (1991). Intention-to-treat policy for analyzing randomized trials: Statistical distortions and neglected clinical challenges, Chapter 28. In *Patient Compliance in Medical Practice and Clinical Trials* (eds. by J.A. Cramer and B. Spilker), Raven Press Ltd, New York.

Finkelstein, D.M. and Schoenfeld, D.A. (1994). Analysing survival in the presence of an auxiliary variable, *Statist. Med.* **13**: 1747–1754.

Finney, D.J. (1990). Repeated Measurements: what is measured and what repeats? *Statist. Med.* **9**: 639–644.

Firth, D. (1987). On the efficiency of quasi-likelihood estimation, *Biometrika* **74**: 233–246.

Fisher, R.A. and MacKenzie, W.A. (1923). Studies in crop variation: II. The manurial response of different potato varieties, *J. Agri. Sci.* **13**: 311–320.

Fitzmaurice, G.M., Laird, N. and Rotnltzky, A. (1993). Regression models for discrete longitudinal responses, *Statist. Sci.* **8**: 284–309.

Fleiss, J.L. (1986). *The Design and Analysis of Clinical Experiments*, Wiley, New York.

Fleiss, J.L. (1993). The statistical basis of meta-analysis, *Statist. Meth. Med. Res.* **2**: 121–145.

Follman, D. (1995). Multivariate tests for multiple endpoints in clinical trials. *Statist. Med.* **14**: 1163–1175.

Fox, W., Sutherland, I. and Daniels, M. (1954). A five-year assessment of patients in a controlled trial of streptomycin in pulmonary tubercolosis, *Quart. J. Med.* **23**: 347.

Freedman, L.S. (1982). Tables of the number of patients required in clinical trials using the logrank test, *Statist. Med.* **1**: 121–130.

Freedman, L.S. and Spiegehalter, D.J. (1983). The assessment of subjective opinion and its use in relation to stopping rules for clinical trials. *The Statist.* **32**: 153–161.

Freedman, L.S., Spiegehalter, D.J. and Parmar, M.K.B. (1994). The what, why and how of Bayesian Clinical trials monitoring, *Statist. Med.* **13**: 1371–1384.

Freidman, L.M., Furberg, C.D. and De Mets, D.L. (1985). *Fundamentals of Clinical Trials*, 2nd ed., PSB Publishing, Littleton, MA.

Freiman, J.A., Chalmers, T.C. and Smith, H. (1978). The importance of beta, the type II error and sample size in the design and interpretation of the randomized control trial: survey of 'negative' trials, *N. Engl. J. Med.* **299**: 690–694.

Freirich, E., Gehan *et al.* (1963). The effect of 6-mercaptopurine on the duration of steroi-induced remissions in acute leukaemia; a model for evaluation of other potentially useful therapies, *Blood* **21**: 699–716.

Frison, L. and Pocock, S.J. (1992). Repeated measures in clinical trials: analysis using mean summary statistics and its implications for design, *Statist. Med.* **11**: 1685–1704.

Gail, M.H. and Simon, R. (1985). Testing for qualitative interactions between treatment effects and patient subsets, *Biometrics* **41**: 361–372.

Gardner, M.J. and Altman, D.G. (1986). Confidence intervals rather than p-values: estimation rather than hypothesis testing, *Br. J. Med.* **292**: 746.

Gardner, M.J. and Altman, D.G. (1989). *Statistics with Confidence*, British Medical Journal, London.

Gehan, E.A. (1984). The evaluation of therapies: Historical control studies, *Statist. Med.* **3**: 315–324.

Gelman, A. (1996). Inference and monitoring convergence. In *Markov Chain Monte Carlo in Practice* (eds. W.R. Gilks, S. Richardson and D.J. Spiegelhalter), Chapman and Hall, London, pp. 131–144.

Giardiello, F.M., Hamilton, S.R., Krush, A.J., Piantadosi, S., Hylind, L.M., Celano, P., Booker, S.V., Robinson, C.R. and Offerhaus, G.J.A. (1993). Treatment of colonic and rectal adenomas with sulindac in familial adenomatous polyposis, *N. Engl. J. Med.* **328**: 1313–1316.

Gilks W.R., Richardson, S. and Spiegelhalter, D.J. (1996). Introducing Markov Chain Monte Carlo. In *Markov Chain Monte Carlo in Practice* (eds. W.R. Gilks, S. Richardson and D.J. Spiegelhalter), Chapman and Hall, London, pp. 1–20.

Gilks, W.R., Clayton, D.G., Spiegelhalter, D.J., Best, N.G., McNeil, A.J., Sharples, L.D. and Kirby, A.J. (1993). Modelling complexity: applications of Gibbs sampling in medicine, *J. Roy. Statist. Soc.* **B55**: 39–52.

Gill, R. and Schumacher, M. (1987). A simple test of the proportional hazards assumption, *Biometrika* **74**: 289–300.

Glonek, G.F.V. and McCullagh, R. (1995). Multivariate logistic models, *J. Roy. Statist. Soc. Ser.* **B57**: 533–546.

Godambe, V.P. (1960). An optimal property of regular maximum likelihood estimation, *Ann. Math. Statist.* **31**: 1209–1211.

Goetghebeur, E.J.T. and Shapiro, S.H. (1996). Analysing non-compliance in clinical trials: Ethical imperative or mission impossible? *Statist. Med.* **15**: 2813–2826.

Goldstein, H. (1991). Nonlinear multilevel models, with an application to discrete response data, *Biometrika* **78**: 45–51.

Gornbein, J.A., Lazaro, C.G. and Little, R.J.A. (1992). Incomplete data in repeated measures analysis, *Statist. Meth. Med. Res.* **I**: 275–295.

Gould, A.L. (1998). Multi-centre trial analysis revisited, *Statist. Med.* **17**: 1779–1797.

Greenwald, A.G. (1975). Consequences of prejudice against the null hypothesis, *Psychol. Bull.* **85**: 845–857.

Grossman, J., Paramar, M.K.B., Spiegelhalter, D.J. and Freedman, L.S. (1994). A unified method for monitoring and analysing controlled trials, *Statist. Med.* **13**: 1815–1826.

Hastle, T.J. and Tibshirani, R.J. (1990). *Generalized Additive Models*, Chapman and Hall, London and New York.

Heart Special Project Committee. (1988). Organization, review and administration of cooperative studies (Greehberg Report): A report from the Heart Special Project Committee to the National Advisory Council, May 1967, *Contr. Clin. Trials* **9**: 137–148.

Hedges, L.V. (1998). Bayesian meta-analysis. In *Statistical Analysis of Medical Data: New Developments* (eds. B. Everitt and G. Dunn), Arnold, New York, pp. 251–276.

Heyting, A., Tolboom, J.T.B.M. and Essers, J.G.A. (1992). Statistical handling of drop-outs in longitudinal clinical trials, *Statist. Med.* **11**: 2043–2061.

Hjalmarson, A., Elmfeldt, D., Herlitz, J., Holmberg, S., Nyberg, G., Ryden, L., Swedberg, K., Waagstein, F., Waldenstram, A., Vedin, A., Wedel, H., Wilhelmsen, L. and Wilhelmsson, C. (1981). A double blind trial of metoprolol in acute myocardial infarction — effects on mortality, *Circulation* **64**: 140.

Hochberg, T. (1988). A sharper Bonferroni procedure for multiple tests of significance, *Biometrika* **75**: 800–803.

Holm, S. (1979). A simple sequentially rejective multiple test procedure. *Scand. J. Statist.* **6**: 65–70.

Holtzman, J.L., Kiam, D.C., Berry, D.C., Mottonen, L., Barrett, G., Harrison, L.I. and Conrard, G.J. (1987). The pharmacodynamic and pharmacokinetic interaction of flecouride acetate and propranolol; effects on cardiac function and drug clearance, *Eur. J. Clin. Pharmacol.* **33**: 97–99.

Hsieh, F.Y., Crowley, J. and Tormey, D.C. (1983). Some test statistics for use in multistate survival analysis, *Biometrika* **70**: 111–119.

Huber, P. (1967). The behaviour of maximum likelihood estimators under nonstandard conditions, *Proc. Fifth Berkeley Symp. Math. Statist. Probab.* 1, 221–233. University of California Press, Berkeley.

ISIS-2 Collaborative Group (1988). Randomized trial of intravenous streptokinase, oral aspirin, both or neither among 17 187 cases of suspected acute myocardial infarction. ISIS-2. *Lancet* **2**: 349–360.

Jennison, C. and Turnbull, B. (1989). Interim analysis: The repeated confidence interval approach (with discussion), *J. Roy. Statist. Soc. Ser.* **B51**: 305–362.

Jones, B. and Kenward, M.G. (1989). *Design and Analysis of Cross-over Trials*, Chapman and Hall, London.

Jones, B., Teather, D., Wang, J. and Lewis, J.A. (1998). A comparison of various estimators of a treatment difference for a multi-centre clinical trial, *Statist. Med.* **17**: 1767–1777.

Kalbfleisch, E.L. and Prentice, R.L. (1973). Marginal likelihood based on Cox's regression and life model, *Biometrika*, **60**: 267–278.

Kalbfleisch, J.D. and Prentice, R.L. (1980). *The Statistical Analysis of Failure Time Data*, Wiley, New York.

Kaplan, E.L. and Meier, P. (1958). Nonparametric estimation from incomplete observation, *J. Am. Statist. Assoc.* **53**: 457–481.

Karim, M.R. (1989). Technical Report #674, Dept. of Biostatistics, John Hopkins University.

Kass, R.E. and Wasserman, L. (1996). The selection of prior distributions by formal rules, *J. Am. Statist. Assoc.* **91**: 1434–1470.

Kenward, M.G. and Jones, B. (1992). Alternative approaches to the analysis of binary and categorical repeated measurements, *J. Blopharmal. Studies* **2**: 137–170.

Kenward, M.G., Lesaffre, E. and Molenberghs, G. (1994). An application of ML and GEE to the analysis of ordinal data from a long study with cases. *Biometrics*, **50**: 945–953.

Kenward, M.G. (1987). A method for comparing profiles of repeated measurements, *Appl. Statist.* **36**: 296–308.

Knatterud, G.L., Rockhold, F.W., George, S.L., Barton, F.B., Davis, C.E., Fairweather, W.R., Honohan, T., Mowery, R. and O'Neill, R. (1998). Guidelines for quality assurance in multicenter trials: A position paper, *Cont. Clin. Trials* **19**: 477–93.

Kuipers, E., Fowler, D., Garety, P., Chisholm, D., Freeman, D., Dunn, G., Bebbington, P. and Hadley, C. (1998). London-East Anglia randomised controlled trial of cognitive-behavioural therapy for psychosis III Follow-up and economic evaluation at 18 months, *Br. J. Psychiat.* **173**: 61–68.

Lagokos, S.W. (1977). Using auxiliary variables for improved estimates of survival time, *Biometrics* **33**: 399–404.

Laird, N.M. (1988). Missing data in longitudinal studies, *Statist. Med.* **7**: 305–315.

Lan, K.K.G. and De Mets, D.L. (1983). Discrete sequential boundaries for clinical trials, *Biometrika* **70**: 659–663.

Lapaucis, A., Sackett, D.L. and Roberts, R. (1988). An assessment of clinically useful measures of the consequences of treatment, *N. Engl. J. Med.* **26**: 1728–1733.

Lavori, P.W. (1992). Clinical trials in psychiatry: Should protocol deviation censor patient data? *Neuropsychopharmacology* **6**: 39–48.

Lee, E.T. (1992). *Statistical Methods for Survival Data Analysis*, Wiley, New York.

Lee, Y.J. (1983). Quick and simple approximations of sample sizes for comparing two independent binomial distributions: Different-sample size case, *Biometrics* **40**: 239–242.

Lee, Y.J., Ellenberg, J.H., Hirtz, D.G. and Nelson, K.B. (1991). Analysis of clinical trials by treatment actually received: is it really and option? *Statist. Med.* **10**: 1595–1605.

Levine, R.J. (1981). *Ethics and Regulations of Clinical Research*, Urban and Schwartzenberg, Baltimore.

Liang, K.-Y. and Zeger. S.L. (1986). Longitudinal data analysis using generalized linear models, *Biometrika*, **73**: 13–22.

Liang, K.-Y., Zeger, S.L. and Qaqish, B. (1992). Multivariate regression analyses for categorical data (with discussion), *J. Roy. Statist. Soc.* **B54**: 3–40.

Lin, D. and Wei, L.J. (1989). The robust inference for the Cox proportional hazards model, *J. Am. Statist. Assoc.* **84**: 1074–1078.

Lind, J. (1753). *A Treatise of the Scurvey reprinted in Lind's Treatise on Scurvey* (eds. C.P. Stewart and D. Guthrie), Edinburgh University Press, Edinburgh, (1953). Sands, Murray, Cochran, Edinburgh.

Lindley, D.V. (1998). Decision analysis and bio-equivalence trials, *Statist. Sci.* **13**: 136–141.

Lindsey, J.K. (1993). *Models for Repeated Measurements*, Oxford Science Publications, Oxford.

Lindsey, J.K. and Lambert, P. (1998). On the appropriateness of marginal models for repeated measurements in clinical trials, *Statist. Med.* **28**: 447–469.

Lipsitz, S.R. and Fitzmaurice, G.M. (1996). Estimating equations for measures of association between repeated binary responses, *Biometrics* **52**: 903–912.

Lipsitz, S.R., Laird, M. and Harrington, D.P. (1991). Generalized estimating equations for correlated binary data: using the odds ratio as a measure of association, *Biometrika* **78**: 153–160.

Lipsitz, S.R., Fitzmaurice, G.M., Orav, E.J. and Laird, N.M. (1994). Performance of generalized estimating equations in practical situations, *Biometrics* **50**: 270–278.

Little, R.J.A. (1995). Modelling the drop-out mechanism in repeated measures studies, *J. Am. Statist. Assoc.* **90**: 1112–1121.

Little, R.J.A. and Rubin, D.B. (1987). *Statistical Analysis with Missing Data*, Wiley, New York.

Louis, T.A., Fienberg, H.V. and Mosteffer, F. (1985). Findings for public health for meta-analysis, *Ann. Rev. Public Health* **6**: 1–20.

Lubsen, J. and Pocock, S.J. (1994). Factorial trials in cardiology: Pros and cons, *Eur. Heart J.* **15**: 585–588.

Machin, D. (1994). Discussions of The What, Why and How of Bayesian Clinical Trials Monitoring, *Statist. Med.* **13**: 1385–1390.

Malmberg, K. (1997). Prospective randomized study of intensive insulin treatment on long term survival after acute myocardial infarction in patients with diabetes mellitus *Br. Med. J.* **314**: 1512–1515.

Mantel, N. and Haenszel, W. (1959). Statistical aspects of the analysis of dates from retrospective studies of disease, *J. Natl. Cancer Inst.* **22**: 719–748.

Marubini, E. and Valsecchi, M.G. (1995). *Analysing Survival Data from Clinical Trials and Observational Studies*, Wiley, New York.

Matthews, J.N.S. (1993). A refinement to the analysis of serial data using summary measures, *Statist. Med.* **12**: 27–37.

Matthews, J.N.S. (1994). Discussion of Diggle and Kenward, *Appl. Statist.* **43**: 49–93.

Matthews, J.N.S., Altman, D.G., Campbell, M.J. and Royston, P. (1989). Analysis of serial measurements in medical research, *Br. Med. J.* **300**: 230–235.

Mauritsen, R.H. (1984). *Logistic regression with random effects*, Unpublished PhD thesis, Department of Biostatistics, University of Washington.

McCullagh, P. (1983). Quasilikelihood functions, *Ann. Statist.* **11**: 59–67.

McCullagh, P. and Nelder, J.A. (1989). *Generalized Linear Models*, 2nd ed., Chapman and Hall, London.

McHugh, R.B. and Lee, C.T. (1984). Confidence estimation and the size of a clinical trial, *Contr. Clin. Trials* **5**: 157–164.

McPherson, K. (1982). On choosing the number of interim analyses in clinical trials, *Statist. Med.* **1**: 25–36.

Medical Research Council. (1931). Clinical trials of new remedies (annotations), *Lancet* **2**: 304.

Meinert, C.L. (1986). *Clinical Trials — Design, Conduct and Analysis*, Oxford University Press, New York.

Meir, P. (1987). Commentary, *Statist. Med.* **6**: 329–331.

Moertel, C.G., Fleming, T.R., MacDonalds and others. (1990). Levamisole and Fluorairacil for adjustment therapy of resected colon carcinoma, *N. Engl. J. Med.* **332**: 353–358.

Moreau, T., O'Quigley, J. and Lellouch, J. (1986). On D. Schoenfeld's approach for testing the proportional hazards assumption, *Biometrika* **73**: 513–515.

Muthen, B.O. (1984). A general structural equation model with dichotomous, ordered categorical and continuous latent variable indicators, *Psychol. Med.* **49**: 115–132.

National Institutes of Health: NIH Almanac. Publication number 81–5, Division of Public Information, Bethesda, MC.

Neale, M.C. (1997). Mx Statistical Modeling. Box 126 MCV, Richmond, VA 23298: Department of Psychiatry. 4th Edition.

Neten, A. and Dennett, J. (1996). Unit Costs of Health and Social Care. Canterbury: Personal Social Services Research Unit, University of Kent.

Normand, S.T. (1999). Meta-analysis: Formulating, evaluating, combining and reporting, *Statist. Med.* **18:** 321–359.

Oakes, M. (1986). *Statistical Inference: A Commentary for the Social and Behavioural Sciences*, John Wiley and Sons, Chichester.

Oakes, M. (1993). The logic and role of meta-analysis in clinical research, *Statist. Meth. Medi. Res.* **2**: 147–160.

O'Brien, P.C. and Fleming, T.R. (1979). A multiple testing procedure for clinical trials, *Biometrics* **35**: 549–556.

Oldham, P.D. (1962). A note on the analysis of repeated measurements of the same subjects, *J. Chron. Dis.* **15**: 969–977.

O'Quigley, J. and Pessione, F. (1989). Score tests for homogeneity of regression effect in the proportional hazards model, *Biometrics* **45**: 135–144.

Pampallona, S. and Tsiatis, A.A. (1994). Group sequential designs for one-sided and two-sided hypothesis testing with provision for early stopping in favour of the null hypothsis, *J. Statist. Plan. Infer.* **42**: 19–35.

Parmar, M.K.B., Spiegelhalter, D.J. and Freedman, L.S. (1994). The CHART trials: design and monitoring, *Statist. Med.* **13**: 1297–1312.

Patterson, H.D., and Thompson, R. (1971). Recovery of inter-block information when block sizes are unequal, *Biometrika* **58**: 545–554.

Patulin Clinical Trials Committee. (1994). Clinical trial of Patulin in the common cold, *Lancet* **2**: 373–375.

Peduzzi, P., Wittes, J. and Detre, K. (1993). Analysis-as-randomized and the problem of nonadherence — an example from the veterans affairs randomized trial of coronory-artery bypass surgery, *Statist. Med.* **12**: 1185–1195.

Persantine-Aspirin Reinfarction Study Research Group (1980). Persantine and aspirin in coronary heart disease, *Circulation* **62**: 449–461.

Peterson, B. and Harrell, F.E. (1990). Partial proportional odds models for ordinal response variables, *Appl. Statist.* **39**: 205–217.

Peto, R. (1982). Statistical aspects of cancer. In *Treatment of Cancer* (ed. K.E. Halnan), Chapman and Hall, London, pp. 867–871.

Peto, R. (1987). Why do we need systematic overviews of randomized trials? *Statist. Med.* **6**: 223–240.

Peto, R., Pike, M.C., Armitage, P. *et al.* (1976). Design and analysis of randomized clinical trials requiring prolonged observation of each patient: I Introduction and Design, *Br. J. Cancer* **34**: 585–612.

Piantadosi, S. (1997). *Clinical Trials: A Methodological Perspective*, Wiley, New York.

Pickles, A.R. (1987). The problem of initial conditions. In *Methods for Longitudinal Data Analysis* (ed. R. Crouchley), Avebury, Aldershot, pp. 129–149.

Pickles, A.R. (1991). The problem of initial condition in longitudinal analysis. In Crouchley, R. (ed.) *Longitudinal Data Analysis*, Aldershot, Averbury, pp. 129–149.

Pickles, A. and Crouchley, R. (1994). Generalizations and applications of frailty models for survival and event data, *Statist. Meth. Med. Res.* **3**: 263–278.

Pickles, A. and Crouchley, R. (1995). A comparison of frailty models for multivariate survival data, *Statist. Med.* **14**: 1447–1461.

Pinheiro, J.C. and De Mets, D.L. (1997). Estimating and reducing bias in group sequential designs with Gaussian independent increment structure, *Biometrika* **84**: 831–845.

Pocock, S.J. (1977). Group sequential methods in the design and analysis of clinical trials, *Biometrika* **62**: 191–199.

Pocock, S.J. (1983). *Clinical Trials*, John Wiley and Sons, Chichester.

Pocock, S.J. (1992). When to stop a clinical trial, *Br. Med. J.* **305**: 235–244.

Pocock, S.J. (1996). Clinical Trials: A statistician's perspective. In *Advances in Biometry* (eds. P. Armitage and H.A. David), Wiley, Chichester.

Pocock, S.J. and Abdalla, M. (1998). The hope and the hazards of using compliance data in randomized controlled trials, *Statist. Med.* **17**: 249–250.

Pocock, S.J., Geller, N.L. and Tsiatis, A.A. (1987). The analysis of multiple end-points in clinical trials, *Biometrics* **43**: 487–498.

Pregibon, D. (1981). Logistic regression diagnostics, *Ann. Statist.* **9**: 705–724.

Prentice, R.L. (1973). Exponential survivals with coronary and explanatory variables, *Biometrika* **60**: 279–288.

Prentice, R.L. (1988). Correlated binary regression with covariates specific to each binary observation, *Biometrics* **44**: 1033–1048.

Prentice, R.L. (1989). Surrogate endpoints in clinical trials: Definitions and operations criteria, *Statist. Med.* **8**: 431–440.

Prentice, R.L. and Zhao, L.P. (1991). Estimating equations for parameters in means and covariances of multivariate discrete and continuous responses, *Biometrics* **47**: 825–883.

Qaqish, B.F. and Liang, K.-Y. (1992). Marginal models for correlated binary responses with multiple classes and multiple levels of nesting, *Biometrics* **48**: 939–950.

Rabe-Hesketh, S. and Everitt, B.S. (1999). The effect of misspecifying the covariance structure when analysing longitudinal data. In preperation.

Reid, N. and Crepeau, H. (1985). Influence functions for proportional hazards regression model. *Biometrika* **72**: 1–9.

Ridout, M. (1991). Testing for random drop-outs in repeated measurement data, *Biometrics* **47**: 1617–1621.

Roberts, G. (1996). Markov chain concepts related to sampling algorithms *Markov Chain Monte Carlo in Practice* (eds. W.R., Gilks, S., Richardson and D.J., Spiegelhalter), Chapman and Hall, London, pp. 45–58.

Robins, J.M. (1998). Correction for non-compliance in equivalence trials, *Statist. Med.* **17**: 269–302.

Robins, J.M. and Rotnitsky, A. (1992). Recovery of information and adjustment for dependent censoring using surrogate markers. In *Aids*

Epidemiology: Methodological Issues (eds. N., Jewell, K., Dietz and V., Farewell), Birkhauser Press.

Robins, J.M., Rotnitzky, A. and Zhao, L.P. (1995). Analysis of semiparametric regression models for repeated outcomes in the presence of missing data, *J. Am. Statist. Assoc.* **90**: 106–121.

Rogers, W.H. (1993). Regression standard errors in clustered samples, *Stata Technical Bulletin* **13**: 19–23. Reprinted in Stata Technical Bulletin Reprints, Vol. 3, pp. 88–94.

Rosner, G. and Tsiatis, A.A. (1989). The impact that group sequential tests would have made on ECOG clinical trials, *Statist. Med.* **8**: 505–516.

Sacks, H.S., Chalmers, T.C. and Smith, H. (1983). Sensitivity and specificity of clinical trials: randomized v's historical controls, *Arch. Inter. Med.* **143**: 753–775.

Sacks, H.S., Chalmers, T.C., Blum, A.L., Berrier, J. and Pagano, D. (1990). Endoscopic hemostasis: an effective therapy for bleeding peptic ulcers, *J. Am. Med. Assoc.* **262**: 494–499.

Sasieni, P. (1993). Maximum weighted partial likelihood estimators for the Cox Model, *J. Am. Statist. Assoc.* **88**: 135–144.

Schluchter, M.D. (1988). Analysis of incomplete multivariate data using linear models with structured covariance matrices, *Statist. Med.* **7**: 317–324.

Schoenfield, D.A. (1980). Chi-squared goodness-of-fit tests for the proportional hazards regression model, *Biometrika* **67**: 145–153.

Schoenfield, D.A. (1982). Partial residues for the proportional hazards regression model, *Biometrika* **69**: 239–241.

Schoenfield, D.A. (1983). Sample size formula for the proportional hazards regression model, *Biometrika* **39**: 499-503.

Schulz, K.F., Chalmers, F., Grimes, D.A. and Altman, D.G. (1994). Assessing the quality of randomization from reports of controlled trials in obstetrics and gynecology journals, *J. Am. Med. Assoc.* **272**: 125–128.

Schwartz, D. and Lellouch, J. (1967). Explanatory and pragmatic attitudes in therapeutic trials, *J. Chron. Disorders* **20**: 637–648.

Segal, M.R. and Neuhaus, J.M. (1993). Robust inference for multivariate survival data. *Statist. Med.* **93**: 1019–31.

Senn, S. (1993). *Cross-over Trials in Clinical Research*, John Wiley and Sons, Chichester.

Senn, S. (1994a). Repeated measures in clinical trials: analysis using mean summary statistics and its implications for design, *Statist. Med.* **13**: 197–198.

Senn, S. (1994b). Testing for baseline balance in clinical trials, *Statist. Med.* **13**: 1715–1726.

Senn, S. (1997). *Statistical Issues in Drug Development*, John Wiley and Sons, Chichester.

Senn, S. (1998). Some controversies in planning and analysing multi-centre trials, *Statist. Med.* **17**: 1753–1765.

Sieh, F.Y. (1987). A simple method of sample size calculation for inequal-sample-size deisgns that use the logrank or t-test, *Statist. Med.* **6**: 577–582.

Silverman, W.A. (1985). *Human Experimentation: A Guided Step into the Unknown*, Oxford Medical Publications, Oxford.

Simon, R. (1982). Randomization and research strategy, *Cancer Treatment Reports* **66**: 1083–1087.

Simon, R. (1991). A decade of progress in statistical methodology for clinical trials, *Statist. Med.* **10**: 1789–1817.

Simon, R. (1994). Some practical aspects of the interim monitoring of clinical trials, *Statist. Med.* **13**: 1401–1409.

Skinner. (1994). Discussion of Diggle and Kenward, *Appl. Statist.* **43**: 49–93.

Smith, D.M. and Diggle, P.J. (1994). OSWALD Version 2: Object Oriented Software for the Analysis of Longitudinal Data in S. Dept. of Mathematics and Statistics, University of Lancaster, England.

Smith, M.L. (1980). Publication bias and meta-analysis, *Eval. Educ.* **4**: 22–24.

Smith, T.C., Spiegelhalter, D.J. and Thomas, A. (1995). Bayesian approaches to random-effects metal-analysis: a comparative study, *Statist. Med.* **14**: 2685–99.

Snell, E.J. (1964). A scaling procedure for ordered categorical data, *Biometrics* **20**: 592–607.

Souhami, R.L. (1994). The clinical importance of early stopping of randomized trials in cancer treatments, *Statist. Med.* **13**: 1293–1295.

Souhami, R.L. and Whitehead, J. (eds.) (1994). Workshop on Early Stopping Rules in Cancer Clinical Trials, *Statist. Med.* **13**: 1289–1500.

Spiegelhalter D. J. Thomas, A., Best, N. and Gilks, W. (1996). BUGS 0.5 Examples. Vol. 1. MRC Biostatistics Unit, Cambridge, England.

Spiegelhalter, D.J., Freedman, L.S. and Parmar, M.K.B. (1994). Bayesian approaches to randomized trials, *J. Roy. Statist. Soc. Ser.* **A157**: 357–416.

Stanley, K.E. (1980). Prognostic factors for survival in patients with inoperable lung cancer. *J. Nat. Cancer Inst.* **65**: 25–32.

Sterlin, T.D. (1959). Publication decisions and their possible effects in inferences drawn from tests of significance — or vice-versa, *J. Am. Statist. Assoc.* **54**: 30–34.

Storer, B.E. and Crowley, J. (1985). A diagnostic for Cox regression and general conditional likelihods. *J. Am. Statist. Assoc.* **80**: 139–147.

Sutton, H.G. (1865). Cases of rheumatic fever, *Guys Hospital Report*, II, pp. 392–428.

Tango, T. (1998). A mixture model to classify individual profiles of repeated measurements. In *Data Science, Classification and Related Methods* (eds. C. Hayashi, N. Oksumi, K. Yajima, Y. Taraka, H.H. Bock and Y. Baba), Springer, Tokyo, pp. 247–254.

Thall, P.F. and Vail, S.C. (1990). Some covariance models for longitudinal count data with overdispersion, *Biometrics* **46**: 657–671.

Therneau, T.M., Grambsch, P.M. and Fleming, T.R. (1990). Martingale hazard regression models and the analysis of censored survival data, *Biometrika* **77**: 147–160.

Thompson, S.G. and Pocock, S.J. (1991). Can meta-analysis be trusted? *Lancet* **338**: 1127–1130.

Thompson, S.G. (1993). Controversies in meta-analysis: the case of the trials of serum cholesterol reduction, *Statist. Meth. Med. Res.* **2**: 173–192.

Troxel, A.B., Fairclough, D.L., Curran, D. and Hahn, E.A. (1998). Statistical analysis of quality of life with missing data in cancer clinical trials, *Statist. Med.* **17**: 653–666.

Tsiatis A.A. (1981). The asymptotic joint distribution of the efficient scores test for the proportional hazards model calculated over time, *Biometrika* **68**: 311–315.

United States Congress. (1962). Drug amendments of 1962, Public Law, 87–781, s1522, Washington.

Urquhart, J. and de Klerk, E. (1998). Contending paradigms for the interpretation of data on patient compliance with therapeutic drug regimes, *Statist. Med.* **17**: 251–268.

Waterhouse, B. (1800). *A Prospect of Exterminating the Small Pox*, Cambridge University Press, Cambridge.

Waterhouse, B. (1802). *A Prospect of Exterminating the Small Pox, Part II*, Cambridge University Press, Cambridge.

Waterhouse, D.M., Calzone, K.A., Mele, C. and Brenner, D.E. (1993). Adherence of oral tamoxifen: A comparison of patient self-report, pill count and microelectronic monitoring, *J. Clin. Oncology* **11**: 1189–1197.

Wedderburn, R.M.W. (1974). Quasilikelihood functions, generalized linear models and the Gauss–Newton method, *Biometrika* **61**: 439–447.

Wei, L.J. and Stram, D.O. (1988). Analying repeated measurements with possibly missing observations by modelling marginal distributions, *Statist. Med.* **7**: 139–148.

White, H. (1980). A heteroskedasticity consistent covariance matrix estimator and a direct test for heteroskedasticity, *Econometrica* **48**: 817–850.

White, H. (1982). Maximum likelihood estimation of misspecified models, *Econometrica* **50**: 1–25.

Whitehead, J. (1986). Sample sizes for phase II and phase III clinical trials, in integrated approach, *Statist. Med.* **5**: 459–464.

Whitehead, J. (1992). *The Design and Analysis of Sequential Clinical Trials*, 2nd ed., Ellis Harwood, New York.

Whitehead, J. (1993). The case for frequentism in clinical trials, *Statist. Med.* **12**: 1405–1415.

Whitehead, J. and Brunier, H. (1995). Bayesian decision procedures for dose determining experiments, *Statist. Med.* **14**: 885–893.

Wild, C.J. and Yee, T.W. (1996). Additive extensions to generalized estimating equations methods, *J. Roy. Statist. Soc.* **B58**: 711–725.

Williams, D.A. (1987). Generalized linear model diagnostics using the deviance and single case deletions, *Appl. Statist.* **36**: 181–191.

Wittes, J. and Wallenstein, S. (1987). The power of the Mantel-Haenszel test, *J. Am. Statist. Assoc.* **82**: 1104–1109.

Wingen, A.M., FabianBach, C., Schaefer, F. and Mehls, O. (1997). Randomized multicentre study of low-protein diet on the progression of chronic renal failure in children, *Lancet* **349**: 1117–1123.

Yates, F. (1982). Regression models for repeated measurements, *Biometrics* **38**: 850–853.

Yusuf, S., Willes, J., Probstfield, J. and Tyroler, H.A. (1991). Analysis and interpretation of treatment effects in subgroups of patients in randomized clinical trials, *J. Am. Med. Assoc.* **266**: 93–98.

Zeger, S.L. and Katz, J. (1998). Graphical presentation of longitudinal data. In *Encyclopedia of Biostatistics* (eds. P. Armitage and T. Colton), Wiley, Chichester.

Zeger, S.L., Liang, K.-Y. and Albert, P.S. (1988). Models for longitudinal data: a generalized estimating equation approach, *Biometrics* **44**: 1049–1060.

Zeger, S.L and Liang, K-Y. (1986). Longitudinal data analysis for discrete and continuous outcomes, *Biometrics* **42**: 121–130.

Zeger, S.L. and Qaqish, B. (1992). Multivariate regression analyses for categorical data (with discussion), *J. Roy. Statist. Soc.* **B54**: 3–40.

Zeger, S.L., Diggle, P.J. and Huang, W. (1998). Generalized linear models for longitudinal data. In *Encyclopedia of Biostatistics* (eds. P. Armitage and T. Cotton), Wiley, Chichester.

Zelen, M. (1983). Guidelines for publishing papers on cancer clinical trials: responsibilities of editors and authors, *J. Clin. Oncol.* **1**: 164–169.

Zhao, L.P. and Prentice, R.L. (1990). Correlated binary regression using a quadratic exponential model, *Biometrika* **77**: 642–648.

Index